365 DAYS OF
AROMATHERAPY

365 Aromatherapy for 365 Days

White Lemon

BOOK NAME

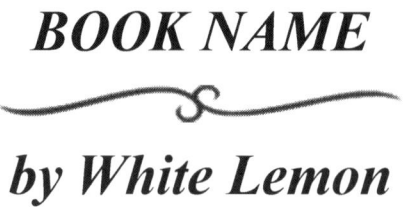

by White Lemon

Copyright © White Lemon 2016

This book is licensed for your personal enjoyment only. This book may not be re-sold or given away to other people. If you would like to share this book with another person, please purchase an additional copy for each recipient. If you're reading this book and did not purchase it, or it was not purchased for your enjoyment only, then please return to your favorite retailer and purchase your own copy. Thank you for respecting the hard work of this author, White Lemon: whitelemon_diy@yahoo.com

See more books by White Lemon:
www.amazon.com/author/whitelemon

Disclaimer

No part of this publication may be reproduced in any form or by any means, including printing, photocopying, or otherwise without prior written permission of the copyright holder. If you would like to use material from the book (other than just simply for reviewing the book), prior permission must be obtained by contacting the author.

ISBN: 978-1539929581

Contents

Introduction 1
    What is Aromatherapy? 3

January 5
    January 1 6
    January 2 6
    January 3 6
    January 4 7
    January 5 7
    January 6 7
    January 7 8
    January 8 8
    January 9 8
    January 10 9
    January 11 9
    January 12 9
    January 13 10
    January 14 10
    January 15 11
    January 16 11
    January 17 11
    January 18 12
    January 19 12
    January 20 12
    January 21 13
    January 22 13
    January 23 13
    January 24 14
    January 25 14
    January 26 14
    January 27 15
    January 28 15
    January 29 16
    January 30 16
    January 31 16

Types of Aromatherapy 17

February 19
    February 1 20
    February 2 20
    February 3 20
    February 4 21
    February 5 21
    February 6 21
    February 7 22
    February 8 22
    February 9 22
    February 10 23

February 11 23
February 12 23
February 13 24
February 14 24
February 15 24
February 16 25
February 17 25
February 18 25
February 19 26
February 20 26
February 21 26
February 22 27
February 23 27
February 24 27
February 25 28
February 26 28
February 27 28
February 28 29
February 29 29

What to Expect from a Cosmetic Aromatherapist 31

March 33

March 1 34
March 2 34
March 3 34
March 4 35
March 5 35
March 6 35
March 7 36
March 8 36
March 9 36
March 10 37
March 11 37
March 12 37
March 13 38
March 14 38
March 15 38
March 16 39
March 17 39
March 18 39
March 19 40
March 20 40
March 21 40
March 22 41
March 23 41
March 24 41
March 25 42
March 26 42
March 27 42
March 28 43
March 29 43
March 30 43
March 31 44

Aromatherapy and Your Pets 45

April 47

    April 1 48
    April 2 48
    April 3 48
    April 4 49
    April 5 49
    April 6 49
    April 7 49
    April 8 50
    April 9 50
    April 10 51
    April 11 51
    April 12 51
    April 13 52
    April 14 52
    April 15 53
    April 15 53
    April 16 53
    April 17 54
    April 18 54
    April 19 54
    April 20 55
    April 21 55
    April 22 55
    April 23 56
    April 24 56
    April 25 56
    April 26 57
    April 27 57
    April 28 57
    April 29 58
    April 30 58

All about Aromatherapy Massage 59

May 61

    May 1 62
    May 2 62
    May 3 62
    May 4 63
    May 5 63
    May 6 63
    May 7 64
    May 8 64
    May 9 64
    May 10 65
    May 11 65
    May 12 65
    May 13 66
    May 14 66
    May 15 66
    May 16 67
    May 17 67

May 18	67
May 19	68
May 20	68
May 21	68
May 22	69
May 23	69
May 24	69
May 25	70
May 26	70
May 27	70
May 28	71
May 29	71
May 30	72
May 31	73

The Benefits of Aromatherapy 75

June 77

June 1	78
June 2	78
June 3	78
June 4	79
June 5	79
June 6	79
June 7	80
June 8	80
June 9	80
June 10	81
June 11	81
June 12	82
June 13	82
June 14	82
June 15	83
June 16	83
June 17	83
June 18	84
June 19	84
June 20	84
June 21	85
June 22	85
June 23	85
June 24	86
June 25	86
June 26	86
June 27	87
June 28	87
June 29	87
June 30	88

Aromatherapy and Children 89

July 91

July 1	92
July 2	92
July 3	92

July 4 93
July 5 93
July 6 93
July 7 94
July 8 94
July 9 94
July 10 95
July 11 95
July 12 95
July 13 96
July 14 96
July 15 97
July 16 97
July 17 97
July 18 98
July 19 98
July 20 98
July 21 99
July 22 99
July 23 99
July 24 100
July 25 100
July 26 100
July 27 101
July 28 101
July 29 101
July 30 102
July 31 102

Types of Aromatherapy Diffusers 103

August 105

August 1 106
August 2 106
August 3 106
August 4 107
August 5 107
August 6 107
August 7 108
August 8 108
August 9 109
August 10 109
August 11 109
August 12 110
August 13 110
August 14 110
August 15 111
August 16 111
August 17 111
August 18 112
August 19 112
August 20 112
August 21 113
August 22 113
August 23 113
August 24 114

August 25 114
August 26 114
August 27 115
August 28 115
August 29 116
August 30 116
August 31 116

Aromatherapy Essential Oil Must-Have's 119

September 121

September 1 122
September 2 122
September 3 122
September 4 123
September 5 123
September 6 123
September 7 124
September 8 124
September 9 124
September 10 125
September 11 125
September 12 125
September 13 126
September 14 126
September 15 126
September 16 127
September 17 127
September 18 127
September 19 128
September 20 128
September 21 128
September 22 129
September 23 129
September 24 130
September 25 130
September 26 130
September 27 131
September 28 131
September 29 131
September 30 132

What You need to Know about Using Essential Oils 133

October 135

October 1 136
October 2 136
October 3 136
October 4 137
October 5 137
October 6 138
October 7 138
October 8 138
October 9 139
October 10 139

October 11 139
October 12 140
October 13 140
October 14 141
October 15 141
October 16 142
October 17 142
October 18 142
October 19 143
October 20 143
October 21 144
October 22 144
October 23 144
October 24 145
October 25 145
October 26 146
October 27 146
October 28 147
October 29 147
October 30 147
October 31 148

How to Use Aromatherapy in Your Bath 149

November 151

November 1 152
November 2 152
November 3 152
November 4 153
November 5 153
November 6 153
November 7 154
November 8 154
November 9 154
November 10 155
November 11 155
November 12 155
November 13 156
November 14 156
November 15 156
November 16 157
November 17 157
November 18 158
November 19 158
November 20 158
November 21 159
November 22 159
November 23 160
November 24 160
November 25 160
November 26 161
November 27 161
November 28 162
November 29 162
November 30 162

Aromatherapy around Your Home 165

December 167

    December 1 168
    December 2 168
    December 3 168
    December 4 169
    December 5 169
    December 6 170
    December 7 170
    December 8 170
    December 9 171
    December 10 171
    December 11 172
    December 12 172
    December 13 172
    December 14 173
    December 15 173
    December 16 174
    December 17 174
    December 18 174
    December 19 175
    December 20 175
    December 21 176
    December 22 176
    December 23 176
    December 24 177
    December 25 177
    December 26 177
    December 27 178
    December 28 178
    December 29 178
    December 30 179
    December 31 179

Conclusion 181

Introduction

We hear about alternative medicines all the time, but how much do we really know about them? For instance, how much do you know about aromatherapy? This is a type of alternative medicine that has been used for centuries to help relieve a number of conditions, from the winter blahs to serious illnesses and then some. While there isn't a lot of science behind aromatherapy, there is evidence that it does indeed work.

Aromatherapy involves using essential oils in combination for the particular problem you are trying to treat. For instance, if you are looking for something to brighten your mood, you will want to use uplifting scents, such as orange and grapefruit. The essential oils used in aromatherapy come from natural sources, including herbs, flowers, and other plants.

There are different ways that you can use aromatherapy treatments. In this e-book, you will find hundreds of recipes for air fresheners, bath products, skin care, hair care, and a whole lot more. You will also find many helpful articles that will help you to learn more about the benefits of using essential oils in aromatherapy, and how to use them.

What is Aromatherapy?

One of the oldest types of holistic healing is aromatherapy. It can help to heal and rejuvenate the body, mind, and soul, and you don't need to use any medications. All you need are scents that smell awesome. Different scents have different effects on the body and mind, and that is basically what aromatherapy is all about. You have probably noticed throughout the years that certain smells trigger certain thoughts and feelings. That is aromatherapy, even if you never realized it

Healing with Scents

Volatile and essential plant oils, or in other words, plant essences, are used to create mixtures that can treat a variety of health issues, from stress to hemorrhoids and everything in between. When used in healing mixtures, the essential oils not only release scents that are pleasing, but they also have healing properties. For instance, peppermint essential oil is great for stomach ailments, and it smells wonderful.

Keep in mind that not all fragrances are beneficial for health purposes, even though they may smell nice. The only fragrances that are actually healthy are those that are natural and come from essential oils. This is because they do not contain any chemicals or other harsh ingredients In fact, all of the recipes in this e-book contain natural ingredients, and other simple ingredients that you probably already have around your home.

Highly Concentrated Scents

When you use essential oils for aromatherapy, you are using highly concentrated scents. This means that a little goes a very long way. You can use essential oils singly, or in combination depending on your reason for using them. The blending of essential oils is known as synergy, and it makes the oils more effective than they are by themselves.

How Aromatherapy Works

When you inhale fragrances, they go through the tiny hairs in your nose, to the part of the brain known as the limbic system. This system is what controls our emotions, moods, and even memory and the ability to learn. When you inhale an aroma, the brain reacts to it, inducing euphoric feelings. This helps you to relax and feel energized.

Certain fragrances can also stimulate love and affection, because they affect our emotions and feelings. Losing one's sense of smell can be extremely detrimental, because it can greatly affect mental and physical health.

Who Uses Aromatherapy?

You have likely heard about people who visit aromatherapists for treatments. Those who use these treatments come from all walks of life. If there is an issue that can be treated through scent, many people are going to try it. In addition to visiting professionals, there are also thousands of recipes you can easily make at home for self-healing. You will find 365 of those recipes here in this e-book.

January

Winter can really wreak havoc on your hair and skin, and this month it is going to start getting a lot colder outside. Luckily, we have loads of recipes this month that use aromatherapy to help your skin stay soft and your hair stay manageable. There are also plenty of great recipes for using diffuser blends so you can enjoy your favorite blends at any time, throughout your home.

January 1

Winter Refresher Diffuser Blend

Materials

- 2 drops grapefruit essential oil
- 3 drops sweet orange essential oil

Directions

Blend oils in your diffuser and use as instructed.

January 2

Beat the Winter Blahs Bath Salts

Materials

- 12 drops bergamot essential oil
- 8 drops clary sage essential oil
- 1 ½ C Epsom salts
- 1 ½ C coarse sea salt

Directions

Combine ingredients together in a glass bowl. Store in a clean jar with a lid. To use, add ½ C to bathwater.

January 3

Pick-Me-Up Bath Oil

Materials

- 2 ounces jojoba oil
- 10 drops orange essential oil
- 8 drops ginger essential oil

Directions

Combine ingredients and store in a dark colored bottle (amber is best as it doesn't allow light in). To use, add ¼ ounce to bathwater.

January 4

Refreshing Massage Oil

Materials

- 1 ounce sweet almond oil
- 6 drops grapefruit essential oil
- 4 drops cypress essential oil

Directions

Mix all ingredients together and store in a dark colored glass bottle. To use, apply ½ tsp per massage.

January 5

Uplifting Diffuser Blend

Materials

- 3 drops bergamot essential oil
- 2 drops clary sage essential oil

Directions

Blend oils in your diffuser and use as instructed.

January 6

Refreshing Diffuser Blend

Materials

- 3 drops bergamot essential oil
- 1 drop neroli essential oil
- 1 drop jasmine essential oil

Directions

Blend oils in your diffuser and use as instructed.

January 7

Aromatherapy Treatment for Dry Hair

Materials

- 1 ounce jojoba oil
- 5 drops sandalwood essential oil
- 3 drops chamomile essential oil
- 2 drops ylang ylang essential oil

Directions

Combine all ingredients in a glass bowl. To use, heat in the microwave, and apply all over hair. You may need to double the recipe if you have long hair. Cover hair with a shower cap or plastic wrap, and let the mixture sit for at least 30 minutes. Rinse, and shampoo as normal.

January 8

More Aromatherapy for Dry Hair

Materials

- 1 ounce raw honey
- ½ ounce jojoba oil
- 1 egg yolk
- 5 drops rosemary essential oil

Directions

Beat the egg yolk and add the honey, jojoba oil, and rosemary essential oil. Wet hair and apply mixture. Cover hair with a shower cap or plastic wrap and let mixture sit for at least 30 minutes. Rinse and wash hair as normal.

January 9

Hair Elixir

Materials

- ½ C pure distilled water
- ½ ounce liquid aloe vera
- 3 drops chamomile essential oil
- 2 drops rosemary essential oil
- 2 drops lavender essential oil

Directions

Mix all ingredients together in a glass bowl. After washing hair, apply mixture before drying. Do not rinse out as this is a leave-in treatment.

January 10

Aromatherapy for Dry Skin

Materials

- 25ml base cream
- 1 tsp wheat germ oil
- 1 tsp rice bran oil
- 4 drops chamomile essential oil
- 3 drops sandalwood essential oil
- 3 drops rose essential oil

Directions

Combine all ingredients together and store in an airtight container. To use, apply to face and neck in the morning and at night.

January 11

Itchy Skin Recipe

Materials

- 100ml witch hazel
- 10 drops lavender essential oil
- 4 drops frankincense essential oil
- 6 drops tea tree oil

Directions

Combine ingredients together in a spray bottle. Shake well before each use.

January 12

Aromatherapy for Brighter Skin

Materials

- 50ml base cream

- 2 tsp wheat germ oil
- 2 tsp hazelnut oil
- 8 drops grapefruit essential oil
- 8 drops mandarin orange essential oil
- 5 drops ylang ylang essential oil

Directions

Combine all ingredients together and store in a dark colored glass bottle. To use, massage a couple of drops into skin once or twice daily.

January 13

Recipe for Chapped Lips

Materials

- 40ml aloe vera gel
- 2 drops chamomile essential oil
- 4 drops geranium essential oil
- 5 drops rose essential oil
- 2 drops neroli essential

Directions

Combine ingredients and store in lip gloss tubs. To use, apply a couple of drops of mixture to dry lips and gently massage.

January 14

Aromatherapy Bath for Colds and Flus

Materials

- 3 drops lavender essential oil
- 2 drops Manuka essential oil
- 1 drop ravensara essential oil

Directions

Combine ingredients and add to bath water.

January 15

Cold and Flu Blend 2

Materials

- 2 drops ravensara essential oil
- 2 drops rosemary essential oil
- 2 drops tea tree oil

Directions

Combine ingredients and add to bath water.

January 16

Sore Throat Bath Blend

Materials

- 3 drops lavender essential oil
- 2 drops thyme essential oil
- 1 drop tea tree oil

Directions

Combine ingredients and add to bath water.

January 17

Cough Blend

Materials

- 2 drops lavender essential oil
- 2 drops sandalwood essential oil
- 2 drops frankincense essential oil

Directions

Combine ingredients and add to bath water.

January 18

Aromatherapy Bath for Tired Muscles

Materials

- 3 drops lavender essential oil
- 2 drops marjoram essential oil
- 1 drop juniper essential oil

Directions

Combine ingredients and add to bath water.

January 19

Tired Muscle Blend 2

Materials

- 3 drops rosemary essential oil
- 2 drops marjoram essential oil
- 1 drop pine essential oil

Directions

Combine ingredients and add to bath water.

January 20

Cracked Skin Blend

Materials

- ½ C unscented skin lotion
- 5 drops patchouli essential oil
- 10 drops sandalwood essential oil
- 2 drops carrot seed essential oil

Directions

Combine all ingredients together and store in an airtight container. To use, rub lotion into affected areas.

January 21

Aromatherapy Dry Skin Body Scrub

Materials

- 1 C Epsom salts
- 1 C coarse sea salt
- 5 drops chamomile essential oil
- 5 drops lavender essential oil
- 3 drops rose essential oil

Directions

Combine all ingredients together in a glass bowl. Transfer to a covered, air-tight container. To use, add ½ of the mixture to bathwater.

January 22

Decongestion Bath Blend

Materials

- 3 drops tea tree oil
- 2 drops thyme essential oil
- 3 drops lavender essential oil
- 2 drops pine essential oil
- 2 drops cinnamon leaf essential oil
- 1 ounce rice bran oil

Directions

Combine ingredients together and store in a dark colored glass bottle. To use, add a few drops to your bathwater.

January 23

Cold and Flu Blend 3

Materials

- 3 drops tea tree oil
- 2 drops lemon myrtle essential oil
- 3 drops lavender essential oil
- 2 drops thyme essential oil
- 1 drop chamomile essential oil
- 1 ounce rice bran oil

Directions

Combine ingredients together and store in a dark colored glass bottle. To use, add a few drops to your bathwater.

January 24

Winter Diffuser Blend

Materials

- 2 drops clove essential oil
- 2 drops sweet orange essential oil
- 1 drop ginger essential oil

Directions

Combine ingredients in your diffuser and use as instructed.

January 25

Uplifting Aromatherapy Body Spray

Materials

- 1 C witch hazel
- 5 drops bergamot essential oil
- 2 drops jasmine essential oil
- 5 drops lemongrass essential oil
- 2 drops neroli essential oil

Directions

Combine all ingredients in a spray bottle. Shake well before each use.

January 26

Aromatic Body Scrub

Materials

- 5 tbsp coarse sea salt
- ½ tsp jojoba oil
- 4 drops peppermint essential oil

Directions

Combine all ingredients together in a glass bowl. Add a few drops of pure distilled water to moisten mixture. Use as you would a regular body scrub.

January 27

Orange Cinnamon Facial Scrub

Materials

- 4 tbsp almond meal
- 1 tsp orange zest
- 1 tbsp natural yogurt
- 2 tbsp raw honey
- ½ tsp ground cinnamon
- 2 drops cinnamon essential oil
- 2 drops sweet orange essential oil

Directions

Combine all ingredients together in a glass bowl. To use, apply all over your face, avoiding your eyes. Rinse with warm water.

January 28

Aromatic Skin Moisturizer

Materials

- 3 tbsp jojoba oil
- 1 tbsp aloe vera gel
- 1 tbsp carrot infused oil
- 8 drops geranium essential oil
- 6 drops lavender essential oil

Directions

Combine all ingredients together in a glass bowl. Use a beater to whip mixture until it begins to thicken. Transfer to a covered glass jar. Shake well before each use as ingredients will separate.

January 29

Aromatherapy Chest Rub for Congestion

Materials

- 2 tbsp avocado oil
- 12 drops naouli essential oil
- 10 drops peppermint essential oil
- 5 drops benzoin essential oil

Directions

Combine all ingredients together in a glass bowl. To use, tub on the chest, throat, and upper back to relieve congestion.

January 30

Eucalyptus Vapor Relief for Congestion

Materials

- 1 liter boiling water
- 5 drops eucalyptus essential oil

Directions

Place eucalyptus essential oil in a bowl with the boiling water. To use, place head over bowl and cover with a towel. Inhale the vapors.

January 31

Digestive Support Blend

Materials

- 10 drops cardamom essential oil
- 10 drops ginger essential oil
- 5 drops tarragon essential oil

Directions

Combine ingredients and store in a dark colored glass bottle. To use, massage onto the skin on your stomach.

Types of Aromatherapy

Now that you know what aromatherapy is used for, it is time to learn about the various types of aromatherapy. It isn't just all about opening a vial of essential oils and inhaling. There are actually three main types of aromatherapy: fragrance; massage/topical application; and cosmetic. Each is used for different purposes, and in some cases, a combination of the different types of aromatherapy is used to treat an illness or other issue. Let's take a look at what is involved with each type of aromatherapy.

Fragrance-Based Aromatherapy

This is a type of aromatherapy that uses only smell for therapeutic treatments. Basically, all you have to do is inhale an essential oil or a combination of essential oils. The olfactory senses are stimulated because the brain is stimulated by the memories of certain scents. Fragrance-based aromatherapy is used to harmonize and regulate the body's natural forces and bring balance to body and mind.

Cosmetic Aromatherapy

This is when essential oils are mixed with other ingredients to create products for skin and hair care. In this e-book, you will find loads of terrific cosmetic aromatherapy recipes for shampoos, hair conditioners, soaps, lotions, scrubs, body butters, and more. This is such a popular form of aromatherapy that may of the biggies in the cosmetics industry are using the science of aromatherapy when creating new skin and hair care products.

Massage or Topical Application Aromatherapy

One of the great things about essential oils is that they are easily absorbed into the skin. This means that they can actually get into your blood stream and offer some serious health benefits. You will enjoy total holistic body healing, because the oils are going to benefit your internal organs. Many essential oils have antifungal properties, anti-viral properties, and antiseptic properties, and can be used to heal a number of issues through massage and the use of topical creams and lotions.

White Lemon

February

February is the month for romance, so naturally we have included a number of awesome recipes for romantic diffuser blends, bath oils, body sprays, and much more. You will also find recipes that you can use to treat many common ailments, and a few household cleaner recipes that will make every room in your home smell like an aromatherapy session.

February 1

Romantic Mood Setter Diffuser Blend 1

Materials

- 2 drops ylang ylang essential oil
- 2 drops patchouli essential oil
- 1 drop black pepper essential oil
- 1 drop ginger essential oil

Directions

Combine ingredients in your diffuser and use as instructed.

February 2

Romantic Mood Setter Diffuser Blend 2

Materials

- 2 drops rose otto essential oil
- 3 drops grapefruit essential oil
- 1 drop sandalwood essential oil
- 1 drop patchouli essential oil

Directions

Combine ingredients in your diffuser and use as instructed.

February 3

Romantic Mood Setter Diffuser Blend 3

Materials

- 2 drops cardamom essential oil
- 2 drops black pepper essential oil
- 2 drops patchouli essential oil

Directions

Combine ingredients in your diffuser and use as instructed.

February 4

Romantic Mood Setter Diffuser Blend 4

Materials

- 2 drops petitgrain essential oil
- 1 drop ylang ylang essential oil
- 1 drop neroli essential oil

Directions

Combine ingredients in your diffuser and use as instructed.

February 5

Romantic Mood Setter Diffuser Blend 5

Materials

- 2 drops bergamot essential oil
- 1 drop jasmine essential oil
- 1 drop sandalwood essential oil

Directions

Combine ingredients in your diffuser and use as instructed.

February 6

Romantic Perfume

Materials

- 1 ounce rice bran oil
- 10 drops rose essential oil
- 10 drops jasmine essential oil
- 10 drops ylang ylang essential oil

Directions

Combine all ingredients together and store in a dark colored glass bottle. To use, dab a bit of mixture onto pulse points.

February 7

Valentine's Day Perfume

Materials

- 1 ounce jojoba oil
- 8 drops sweet orange essential oil
- 8 drops neroli essential oil
- 8 drops ginger essential oil
- 2 drops black pepper essential oil.

Directions

Combine all ingredients together and store in a dark colored glass bottle. To use, dab a bit of mixture onto pulse points.

February 8

Lovers' Perfume

Materials

- 1 ounce rice bran oil
- 8 drops rose essential oil
- 4 drops sandalwood essential oil

Directions

Combine all ingredients together and store in a dark colored glass bottle. To use, dab a bit of mixture onto pulse points.

February 9

Aromatic Milk Bath for Soft Skin 1

Materials

- 1C whole milk
- 2 drops clove essential oil
- 2 drops cinnamon essential oil
- 1 drop ginger essential oil

Directions

Combine ingredients together and add to bath water.

February 10

Aromatic Milk Bath for Soft Skin 2

Materials

- 1C whole milk
- 3 drops jasmine essential oil
- 2 drops ylang ylang essential oil

Directions

Combine ingredients together and add to bath water.

February 11

Seductive Bath Salts

Materials

- ½ C Epsom salts
- ½ C coarse sea salt
- 5 drops ginger essential oil
- 5 drops ylang ylang essential oil
- 5 drops vanilla essential oil

Directions

Combine ingredients together in a glass bowl. Transfer to a covered, airtight container. To use, add ½ C of the mixture to your bathwater.

February 12

Romantic Massage Butter

Materials

- 2 ounces cocoa butter
- 2 ounces coconut oil
- 7 drops rose essential oil
- 3 drops lavender essential oil

Directions

In a double boiler over medium heat, melt the cocoa butter and coconut oil. Remove from heat and add essential oils. To use, warm in your hands and apply while massaging.

February 13

In the Mood Diffuser Blend 1

Materials

- 3 drops grapefruit essential oil
- 1 drop rose essential oil
- 1 drop patchouli essential oil
- 1 drop sandalwood essential oil

Directions

Combine ingredients in your diffuser and use as instructed.

February 14

In the Mood Diffuser Blend 2

Materials

- 2 drops petitgrain essential oil
- 1 drop neroli essential oil
- 1 drop ylang ylang essential oil

Directions

Combine ingredients in your diffuser and use as instructed.

February 15

In the Mood Diffuser Blend 3

Materials

- 2 drops bergamot essential oil
- 1 drop jasmine essential oil
- 1 drop sandalwood essential oil

Directions

Combine ingredients in your diffuser and use as instructed.

February 16

In the Mood Diffuser Blend 4

Materials

- 2 drops lavender essential oil
- 2 drops lemon essential oil
- 1 drop tuberose essential oil

Directions

Combine ingredients in your diffuser and use as instructed.

February 17

In the Mood Diffuser Blend 5

Materials

- 2 drops frankincense essential oil
- 2 drops mandarin orange essential oil
- 1 drop jasmine essential oil

Directions

Combine ingredients in your diffuser and use as instructed.

February 18

Focus Diffuser Blend

Materials

- 2 drops peppermint essential oil
- 2 drops orange essential oil

Directions

Combine ingredients in your diffuser and use as instructed.

February 19

Fresh Smelling Diffuser Blend

Materials

- 2 drops rosemary essential oil
- 2 drops lavender essential oil
- 2 drops lemon essential oil

Directions

Combine ingredients in your diffuser and use as instructed.

February 20

Odor Eliminating Diffuser Blend

Materials

- 2 drops lemon essential oil
- 1 drop lime essential oil
- 1 drop grapefruit essential oil
- 1 drop orange essential oil
- 1 drop cilantro essential oil

Directions

Combine ingredients in your diffuser and use as instructed.

February 21

Clear Breathing Diffuser Blend

Materials

- 2 drops lemon essential oil
- 2 drops lavender essential oil
- 2 drops peppermint essential oil

Directions

Combine ingredients in your diffuser and use as instructed.

February 22

Citrus Diffuser Blend

Materials

- 2 drops sweet orange essential oil
- 1 drop grapefruit essential oil
- 2 drops lime essential oil
- 2 drops lemon essential oil

Directions

Combine ingredients in your diffuser and use as instructed.

February 23

Meditation Diffuser Blend

Materials

- 1 drop ylang ylang essential oil
- 1 drop bergamot essential oil
- 1 drop patchouli essential oil

Directions

Combine ingredients in your diffuser and use as instructed.

February 24

Respirator Diffuser Blend

Materials

- 2 drops peppermint essential oil
- 1 drop eucalyptus essential oil
- 1 drop lemon essential oil
- 1 drop rosemary essential oil

Directions

Combine ingredients in your diffuser and use as instructed.

February 25

Aromatherapy Dish Liquid

Materials

- 2 C liquid Castile soap
- 4 drops lemon essential oil
- 3 drops orange essential oil

Directions

Combine all ingredients together. Transfer to an empty dish liquid bottle and use as you would regular dish liquid.

February 26

Aromatic Room Spray

Materials

- 1 C pure distilled water
- 5 drops peppermint essential oil
- 2 drops pine essential oil
- 2 drops eucalyptus essential oil

Directions

Combine all ingredients together in a glass bowl. Transfer to a spray bottle. Shake well before each use.

February 27

Man-Cave Diffuser Blend

Materials

- 2 drops wintergreen essential oil
- 2 drops peppermint essential oil
- 2 drops spearmint essential oil
- 1 drop cypress essential oil

Directions

Combine ingredients in your diffuser and use as instructed.

February 28

Citrus Spice Diffuser Blend

Materials

- 3 drops sweet orange essential oil
- 2 drops cinnamon essential oil
- 2 drops clove essential oil

Directions

Combine ingredients in your diffuser and use as instructed.

February 29

Immunity Boosting Diffuser Blend

Materials

- 1 drop eucalyptus essential oil
- 1 drop rosemary essential oil
- 1 drop cinnamon bark essential oil
- 1 drop clove essential oil
- 1 drop sweet orange essential oil

Directions

Combine ingredients in your diffuser and use as instructed.

What to Expect from a Cosmetic Aromatherapist

If you are interested in cosmetic aromatherapy, you may consider visiting a cosmetic aromatherapist. This is a person who works with essential oils to create cosmetic products that can help treat acne, dry or oily skin, dry or oily hair, dandruff, eczema, and a whole lot more. The cosmetic aromatherapist is someone who is trained in the art and science of aromatherapy, as well as the use of other healthy ingredients for skin and hair care.

Where do Cosmetic Aromatherapists Work?

There are many places where you can find a cosmetic aromatherapist at work. For instance, some set up businesses in their own homes. Others work at beauty salons and spas. Others even work with some medical practices that combine traditional and holistic healing methods. They are able to perform massages and facials, as well as a variety of other natural beauty treatments.

Some cosmetic aromatherapists even create their own line of aromatherapy skin and hair care products. They use combinations of essential oils, carrier oils, and other natural ingredients to create products that are all-natural and healthy. Blends can include facial blends, body blends, foot blends, bath blends, shampoo blends, and more.

It Takes Practice

If you are interested in becoming a cosmetic aromatherapist, you are going to have to do a lot of work. You don't necessarily need to take college courses, but you will need to learn about how certain items react when mixed, scent combinations, etc. There is a lot of trial and error involved in this line of work until you are used to it. The recipes in this e-book will help you get started with the basics if this is a career field you wish to pursue.

March

Spring is just around the corner, so it's time to start making your home smell spring-fresh. We have some great room scent recipes this month that will not only make your home smell great, but will also help with numerous ailments and other issues. You will also find a lot of recipes for diffuser blends, as well as skin and hair care recipes.

March 1

Stress Relief Diffuser Blend

Materials

- 2 drops bergamot essential oil
- 2 drops frankincense essential oil

Directions

Combine ingredients in your diffuser and use as instructed.

March 2

Sleepy Time Diffuser Blend

Materials

- 2 drops chamomile essential oil
- 2 drops lavender essential oil
- 2 drops vetiver essential oil

Directions

Combine ingredients in your diffuser and use as instructed.

March 3

Chill Out Diffuser Blend

Materials

- 2 drops cedarwood essential oil
- 2 drops vetiver essential oil
- 1 drop orange essential oil

Directions

Combine ingredients in your diffuser and use as instructed.

March 4

Rose Bath Salts

Materials

- 1 C Epsom salts
- 1 C coarse sea salt
- 1 tsp rose geranium essential oil
- 4 tbsp finely ground rose petals

Directions

Mix ingredients well and store in an airtight container. To use, add ½ cup of the mixture to your bathwater.

March 5

Romance Bath Bomb

Materials

- 1 ½ C Baking soda
- ½ C citric acid
- 2 tbsp witch hazel
- 3 drops rose essential oil
- 2 drops lavender essential oil

Directions

Mix the baking soda and citric acid. Add the essential oils, and spritz with witch hazel. Pack mixture into molds and allow to dry for 24 hours. To use, add one bomb to your bathwater.

March 6

Peace of Mind Diffuser Blend 1

Materials

- 5 drops lime essential oil
- 3 drops jasmine essential oil
- 1 drop lemon essential oil
- 1 drop cinnamon essential oil

Directions

Combine ingredients in your diffuser and use as instructed.

March 7

Peace of Mind Diffuser Blend 2

Materials

- 12 drops patchouli essential oil
- 5 drops vanilla essential oil
- 2 drops linden blossom essential oil
- 1 drop neroli essential oil

Directions

Combine ingredients in your diffuser and use as instructed.

March 8

Peace of Mind Diffuser Blend 3

Materials

- 4 drops bergamot essential oil
- 3 drops sandalwood essential oil
- 2 drops grapefruit essential oil
- 1 drop jasmine essential oil

Directions

Combine ingredients in your diffuser and use as instructed.

March 9

Peace of Mind Diffuser Blend 4

Materials

- 10 drops lime essential oil
- 7 drops bergamot essential oil
- 2 drops ylang ylang essential oil
- 1 drop rose essential oil

Directions

Combine ingredients in your diffuser and use as instructed.

March 10

Peace of Mind Diffuser Blend 5

Materials

- 4 drops bergamot essential oil
- 2 drops ylang ylang essential oil
- 2 drops grapefruit essential oi
- 2 drops lemon essential oil

Directions

Combine ingredients in your diffuser and use as instructed.

March 11

Relaxation Diffuser Blend 1

Materials

- 5 drops spruce essential oil
- 2 drops cedar essential oil
- 2 drops pine essential oil

Directions

Combine ingredients in your diffuser and use as instructed.

March 12

Relaxation Diffuser Blend 2

Materials

- 5 drops lavender essential oil
- 4 drops rosewood essential oi
- 2 drops ylang ylang essential oil

Directions

Combine ingredients in your diffuser and use as instructed.

March 13

Relaxation Diffuser Blend 3

Materials

- 5 drops rosemary essential oil
- 3 drops lavender essential oil
- 1 drop chamomile essential oil
- 1 drop peppermint essential oil

Directions

Combine ingredients in your diffuser and use as instructed.

March 14

Relaxation Diffuser Blend 4

Materials

- 11 drops lemon essential oil
- 5 drops bergamot essential oil
- 3 drops spearmint essential oil

Directions

Combine ingredients in your diffuser and use as instructed.

March 15

Relaxation Diffuser Blend 5

Materials

- 5 drops bergamot essential oil
- 5 drops lavender essential oil
- 2 drops cypress essential oil

Directions

Combine ingredients in your diffuser and use as instructed.

March 16

Emotional Well-Being Diffuser Blend 1

Materials

- 9 drops orange essential oil
- 5 drops spearmint essential oil
- 3 drops lavender essential oil

Directions

Combine ingredients in your diffuser and use as instructed.

March 17

Emotional Well-Being Diffuser Blend 2

Materials

- 5 drops sandalwood essential oil
- 2 drops lemon essential oil
- 1 drop pine essential oil
- 1 drop rose essential oil

Directions

Combine ingredients in your diffuser and use as instructed.

March 18

Emotional Well-Being Diffuser Blend 3

Materials

- 6 drops orange essential oil
- 2 drops patchouli essential oil
- 2 drops lemon essential oil

Directions

Combine ingredients in your diffuser and use as instructed.

March 19

Emotional Well-Being Diffuser Blend 4

Materials

- 4 drops ylang ylang essential oil
- 4 drops clary sage essential oil
- 3 drops bergamot essential oil

Directions

Combine ingredients in your diffuser and use as instructed.

March 20

Emotional Well-Being Diffuser Blend 5

Materials

- 7 drops sweet orange essential oil
- 3 drops vanilla essential oil
- 2 drops ylang ylang essential oil

Directions

Combine ingredients in your diffuser and use as instructed.

March 21

Emotional Well-Being Diffuser Blend 6

Materials

- 5 drops juniper essential oil
- 4 drops sweet orange essential oil
- 1 drop ylang ylang essential oil

Directions

Combine ingredients in your diffuser and use as instructed.

March 22

Emotional Well-Being Diffuser Blend 7

Materials

- 10 drops sandalwood essential oil
- 2 drops neroli essential oil

Directions

Combine ingredients in your diffuser and use as instructed.

March 23

Aromatherapy Peppermint Foot Scrub

Materials

- 4 tbsp coarse sea salt
- 2 tbsp rice bran oil
- 8 drops peppermint essential oil
- 2 drops tea tree oil

Directions

Mix ingredients together to form a paste. To use, apply to the feet and massage into skin. Rinse with warm water.

March 24

Lemon Peppermint Itchy Feet Scrub

Materials

- ¼ C finely ground oatmeal/cornmeal mix
- 1 tbsp coarse sea salt
- 4 drops peppermint essential oil
- 2 drops lemon essential oil

Directions

Mix ingredients together to form a paste. To use, apply to the feet and massage into skin. Rinse with warm water.

March 25

Aromatherapy Foot Lotion

Materials

- 1 tbsp jojoba oil
- 1 tbsp extra virgin olive oil
- 1 tbsp wheat germ oil
- 8 drops eucalyptus essential oil
- 2 drops peppermint essential oil

Directions

Combine all ingredients and transfer to a dark colored glass bottle. To use, rub a few drops into your feet.

March 26

Aromatherapy Foot Powder

Materials

- 2 tbsp arrowroot powder
- 2 drops rosemary essential oil
- 2 drops tea tree oil

Directions

Mix ingredients together in a glass bowl. To use, dust onto feet and inside socks before putting socks on.

March 27

Aromatherapy for Healthy Nails

Materials

- 1 vitamin E capsule
- 2 drops each: lavender, lemon, patchouli, sandalwood, and tea tree essential oils

Directions

Mix all ingredients together and store in a dark colored glass bottle. To use, apply a couple of drops to each nail and massage.

March 28

Aromatherapy Lotion for Dry Hands

Materials

- 2 tbsp almond oil
- 1 tsp grated beeswax
- 1 tsp shea butter
- 3 drops peppermint essential oil
- 4 drops chamomile essential oil
- 5 drops lemongrass essential oil

Directions

In a double boiler over medium heat, combine beeswax, almond oil, and shea butter. When ingredients have melted and blended together, remove from heat and add essential oils. Pour mixture into a glass jar and allow to cool and harden. To use, apply to hands before bedtime.

March 29

Aromatherapy Facial Mask 1

Materials

- 1 large fresh strawberry
- 1 tbsp plain yogurt
- 1 tsp bentonite clay
- 2 drops lavender essential oil
- 1 drop rosemary essential oil

Directions

Combine all of the ingredients in a glass bowl. To use, apply all over face, avoiding the eyes. Let mask sit for 20 minutes, and rinse with warm water.

March 30

Aromatherapy Facial Mask 2

Materials

- 2 tbsp raw honey
- 3 drops lavender essential oil

Directions

Combine honey and lavender essential oil. To use, apply all over face, avoiding the eyes. Let mask sit for 20 minutes, and rinse with warm water.

March 31

Aromatherapy Body Spray

Materials

- 1 C pure distilled water
- ½ C witch hazel
- 3 drops frankincense essential oil
- 2 drops rose essential oil

Directions

Combine ingredients together in a spray bottle. Shake well before each use.

Aromatherapy and Your Pets

When used properly, aromatherapy can be a great thing for your pets as well as for the human members of your family. While it is of the utmost importance to see a veterinarian when your pets are sick or injured, there are some things you can do to help through the use of aromatherapy. It is important to speak with your vet before using any essential oils, because some can be dangerous to pets. Here, we are going to discuss some of the best essential oils to use for pets, and what safety considerations you need to take when treating your pets with aromatherapy.

Essential Oils for Pets

There are several essential oils that can be safely used in pet care. For instance, lavender has long been used, pure and diluted, to help treat allergies, ulcers, burns, car anxiety, and even car sickness. Other essential oils that are healthy for pets include:

- Frankincense – This essential oil has been known to be helpful in the treatment of certain cancers. It works with the immune system, and can be used to help reduce tumors. It also helps to increase the supply of blood to the brain. Be cautious with frankincense, because too much can lead to hypertension.
- Fennel – This essential oil can help break down toxins and fluid in bodily tissues. It also helps to keep the pituitary, thyroid, and pineal glands balanced.
- Helichrysum – This essential oil has anti-bacterial properties, and can be used to treat infections. It is also used for skin regeneration, and it can even help to repair damaged nerves. It can slow bleeding if your pet has been in an accident. Helichrysum is often used in the treatment of cardiac disease.
- Spearmint – If your pet is overweight, this is a great essential oil to use. It is good for the treatment of coughs, nausea, and diarrhea. It can help to stimulate the gallbladder and help to boost metabolism. It is particularly helpful for cats that have gastrointestinal problems.
- Cardamom – Here is an essential oil that can be used as an anti-bacterial, and it is also used to help normalize the appetite. It can be used to treat colic, coughs, nausea, and heartburn.

Safety Considerations

Essential oils are extremely powerful, and should never be used in their undiluted forms, especially when used on pets. Too much of certain essential oils can actually have negative effects rather than positive ones. Be sure that you are only using therapeutic-grade essential oils, and that you only buy your oils from reputable companies that sell quality oils. Oils should also be diluted to protect your pets' sense of smell. They can smell a lot more than we can, so remember, a tiny bit goes a very long way. It is best to talk with your vet to come up with the best dosage for your pets.

April

Spring has finally sprung, and it's time to open those windows and let the fresh scent of the outdoor air inside. It's also a good time to work on some awesome aromatherapy recipes. This month, we have recipes for spring-fresh diffuser blends, aromatherapy lip balms, skin care items, aromatherapy for your hair, and a whole lot more.

April 1

Aromatherapy Lip Balm

Materials

- 1 tbsp grated beeswax
- ½ tsp rice bran oil
- 2 drops peppermint essential oil

Directions

In a small glass bowl, melt the beeswax in the microwave in 30-second increments. It should be almost melted so it isn't too hot. You can stir it up to get it to completely melt. Add the rice bran oil and peppermint essential oil. Pour into prepared lip balm tub or tube.

April 2

Aromatherapy Bath Salts

Materials

- 1 C Epsom salts
- 1 C coarse sea salt
- 5 drops lemon essential oil
- Yellow food grade colorant (optional)

Directions

Mix all ingredients together in a glass bowl. Transfer to an airtight container. To use, add ½ C of the mixture to your bathwater.

April 3

Skin Refreshing Mud Mask

Materials

- 3 tbsp kaolin clay powder
- 1 tbsp liquid aloe vera
- 2 drops peppermint essential oil
- Liquid from 1 vitamin E capsule

Directions

Combine ingredients together in a glass bowl. Apply all over face, avoiding your eyes. Let sit for 20 minutes and rinse with clear, warm water.

April 4

Spring Fresh Diffuser Blend

Materials

- 3 drops lemon essential oil
- 1 drop pine essential oil

Directions

Combine ingredients in your diffuser and use as instructed.

April 5

Sunny Day Diffuser Blend

Materials

- 3 drops sweet orange essential oil
- 1 drop grapefruit essential oil

Directions

Combine ingredients in your diffuser and use as instructed.

April 6

Lemon Fresh Dish Liquid

Materials

- 2 C liquid Castile soap
- 15 drops lemon essential oil

Directions

Combine ingredients in a clean dish liquid bottle. Use the same way as regular dish liquid.

April 7

Lemon Peppermint Body Spritz

Materials

- 2 C pure distilled water

- Juice from 1 lemon
- 3 drops peppermint essential oil

Directions

Combine ingredients and transfer to a spray bottle. Spritz when you need a pick-me-up.

April 8

Relaxing Bath Oil

Materials

- 2 ounces rice bran oil
- 5 drops sweet orange essential oil
- 3 drops cedarwood essential oil
- 3 drops ylang ylang essential oil

Directions

Combine all of the ingredients in a glass bowl, and pour under the running water in the tub to help it disperse throughout the water better.

April 9

Aromatherapy Soap

Materials

- 1 pound clear glycerin melt and pour soap base
- 8 drops peppermint essential oil
- 10 drops orange essential oil
- Soap molds
- Food-grade colorant (optional)

Directions

In a double boiler over medium heat, melt the soap base. Remove from heat and add the essential oils and colorant if you are using it. Pour mixture into molds and allow to set. If you put the molds into the freezer, the soap will be ready to use in about 20 minutes.

April 10

Aromatherapy Neck Wrap

Materials

- 2 C hot water
- 2 drops lavender essential oil
- 2 drops bergamot essential oil
- 2 drops peppermint essential oil
- Flannel fabric

Directions

Combine all ingredients in a glass bowl. Soak the fabric in the mixture, and wrap it around your neck. Remove before it gets cold.

April 11

Aromatherapy Shampoo for Dry Hair

Materials

- 1 C liquid Castile soap
- 2 tbsp rice bran oil
- 10 drops chamomile essential oil
- 8 drops neroli essential oil

Directions

Combine all ingredients together in a glass bowl. Transfer to a clean shampoo bottle and use as regular shampoo.

April 12

Aromatherapy Shampoo for Oily Hair

Materials

- 1 C liquid Castile soap
- 2 tbsp rice bran oil
- 10 drops lemon essential oil
- 8 drops geranium essential oil

Directions

Combine all ingredients together in a glass bowl. Transfer to a clean shampoo bottle and use as regular shampoo.

April 13

Aromatherapy Shampoo for Normal Hair

Materials

- 1 C liquid Castile soap
- 2 tbsp rice bran oil
- 7 drops lemon essential oil
- 7 drops geranium essential oil
- 7 drops rosemary essential oil

Directions

Combine all ingredients together in a glass bowl. Transfer to a clean shampoo bottle and use as regular shampoo.

April 14

Aromatherapy Shampoo for Dandruff

Materials

- 1 C liquid Castile soap
- 2 tbsp rice bran oil
- 8 drops geranium essential oil
- 8 drops lemon essential oil
- 8 drops rosemary essential oil

Directions

Combine all ingredients together in a glass bowl. Transfer to a clean shampoo bottle and use as regular shampoo.

April 15

Aromatherapy Spot Treatment for Acne

Materials

- 1 ounce kukui nut
- 15 drops lavender essential oil
- 8 drops tea tree oil
- 5 drops cypress essential oil
- 4 drops helichrysum essential oil

Directions

Combine ingredients together in a glass bowl. Transfer to an airtight container for storage. To use, apply to affected areas once or twice daily.

April 15

Aromatherapy Facial Steam for Acne

Materials

- Bowl of steaming hot water
- 1 drop clary sage essential oil
- 1 drop palmarosa essential oil

Directions

Add essential oils to steaming water. Lean over bowl with a towel over your head for five minutes to let the steam do its work and open the pores to make cleansing easier.

April 16

Aromatherapy Facial Mask for Acne

Materials

- 1 tsp kaolin clay
- 1 tsp raw honey
- 1 drop rosemary essential oil
- 1 drop helichrysum essential oil

Directions

Combine ingredients together in a glass bowl. To use, apply all over face, avoiding the eyes. Leave on for 10 minutes, and rinse with clear, warm water.

April 17

Aromatherapy Scalp Refresher

Materials

- ½ ounce sweet almond oil
- 2 drops tea tree oil
- 2 drops lavender essential oil
- 2 drops jasmine essential oil
- 1 drop clary sage essential oil

Directions

Combine all ingredients together and massage into scalp just before rinsing hair.

April 18

Aromatherapy Hair Conditioner

Materials

- ½ ounce jojoba oil
- 2 drops lavender essential oil
- 2 drops sandalwood essential oil
- 2 drops chamomile essential oil
- 1 drop jasmine essential oil

Directions

Combine all ingredients together and use as you would a regular conditioner. Leave in for at least two minutes for deep conditioning.

April 19

Aromatherapy for Dandruff Prevention

Materials

- ½ ounce rice bran oil
- 2 drops tea tree oil
- 2 drops lavender essential oil
- 2 drops ylang ylang essential oil
- 2 drops rosemary essential oil

Directions

Combine ingredients together and massage into the scalp. Cover head with a shower cap, and let mixture sit for at least an hour. Add shampoo and rinse thoroughly.

April 20

Aromatherapy Body Butter

Materials

- ½ C cocoa butter
- 1 C coconut oil
- 2 drops rosemary essential oil
- 2 drops lavender essential oil

Directions

In a double boiler over medium heat, combine the cocoa butter and coconut oil until they have melted and blended together. Remove from heat and add the essential oils. Store in a covered container.

April 21

Orange Air Freshener

Materials

- ½ C pure distilled water
- 25 drops orange essential oil
- 5 drops ylang ylang essential oil
- 10 drops bergamot essential oil
- 3 drops rose essential oil

Directions

Combine all ingredients together in a spray bottle. Shake well before each use.

April 22

Joy Air Freshener

Materials

- ½ C pure distilled water
- 10 drops lemon essential oil

- 8 drops lavender essential oil
- 12 drops clary sage essential oil

Directions

Combine all ingredients together in a spray bottle. Shake well before each use.

April 23

Minty Fresh Air Spray

Materials

- ½ C pure distilled water
- 20 drops spearmint essential oil
- 10 drops peppermint essential oil

Directions

Combine all ingredients together in a spray bottle. Shake well before each use.

April 24

Room Disinfectant Spray

Materials

- ½ C pure distilled water
- 40 drops tea tree oil
- 25 drops thyme essential oil
- 30 drops eucalyptus essential oil

Directions

Combine all ingredients together in a spray bottle. Shake well before each use.

April 25

Room Deodorizing Spray

Materials

- ½ C pure distilled water
- 15 drops bergamot essential oil
- 3 drops eucalyptus essential oil
- 5 drops lemon essential oil

Directions

Combine all ingredients together in a spray bottle. Shake well before each use.

April 26

Citrus Air Freshener

Materials

- ½ C pure distilled water
- 15 drops grapefruit essential oil
- 10 drops lemon essential oil
- 10 drops orange essential oil

Directions

Combine all ingredients together in a spray bottle. Shake well before each use.

April 27

Aromatherapy Massage Oil for Good Sleep

Materials

- 1 ounce rice bran oil
- 6 drops chamomile essential oil
- 4 drops peppermint essential oil
- 3 drops marjoram essential oil

Directions

Combine ingredients together in a glass bowl. To use massage into skin with fingertips.

April 28

Aromatherapy Massage Oil for Cold Relief

Materials

- 1 ounce rice bran oil
- 5 drops lavender essential oil
- 4 drops eucalyptus essential oil
- 4 drops tea tree oil

Directions

Combine ingredients together in a glass bowl. To use massage into skin with fingertips.

April 29

Aromatherapy Massage Oil for Stress Relief

Materials

- 1 ounce rice bran oil
- 7 drops lavender essential oil
- 5 drops chamomile essential oil
- 3 drops petitgrain essential oil

Directions

Combine ingredients together in a glass bowl. To use massage into skin with fingertips.

April 30

Aromatherapy Massage Oil for PMS Relief

Materials

- ½ ounce rice bran oil
- 5 drops marjoram essential oil
- 5 drops clary sage essential oil
- 4 drops ylang ylang essential oil

Directions

Combine ingredients together in a glass bowl. To use massage into skin with fingertips.

All about Aromatherapy Massage

Who doesn't love a good massage? Now, picture a great massage with great scents to go along with it. That is your aromatherapy massage. Highly concentrated essential oils are added to oils and lotions, or used to make oils and lotions for various types of massages. Not only is the massage going to help your aching muscles, the scents will help to lower your heart rate and blood pressure, regulate your breathing, improve your memory, improve your digestion, and improve your immune system.

Skin Absorption for Better Healing

Essential oils are absorbed into the skin, so it only makes sense that they are used in massage therapy. They have a variety of healing properties, and combinations of essential oils can be used to treat various illnesses and other issues through massage. Some of these essential oils are calming, such as chamomile, lavender, and geranium. Others are more uplifting, such as clary sage, rose, and neroli. Some essential oils such as rosemary are used for energizing and cleansing the system, while others like eucalyptus can be used to help clear congestion.

Why is Aromatherapy Massage Used?

There are several reasons why people choose to have aromatherapy massage. It can be used to treat such conditions as insomnia, stress, headaches and migraines, digestive issues, PMS, back pain, and more. It can help those who have lymphedema, and many mothers claim it has helped them to get through post-partum depression. It is also used in the treatment of certain cancers, often in palliative care settings.

What to Expect

You may or may not actually have a massage on your first visit to the aromatherapy massage therapist. The first step of the process is a consultation. They will sit down with you and discuss your reasons for wanting aromatherapy massage. They will tell you the benefits and dangers involved, and look at your health history to make sure that they are using the proper essential oils. If you have any scent allergies, now is the time to let the massage therapist know.

Following the consultation, the massage therapy will begin. Certain essential oils are chosen based on your particular health condition, and blended just for you. This blend is recorded, so it can be repeated for every massage session you have. In addition to having a healing massage, you also get to enjoy a blend of scents that will help you to relax and feel great. You may also be given an essential oil blend to use at home between professional massages.

Precautions

Aromatherapy massage is not always the best form of treatment for everyone. If you have a rash, an open would, or an infectious skin disease, massage is not recommended. It should also not be done immediately after a surgical procedure, or after chemo and radiation treatments unless your doctor recommends it. If you are prone to blood clots, your physician may advise against massage therapy as it can dislodge the clot. Always speak with your doctor before beginning any type of holistic treatments, including aromatherapy massage.

May

This is the best time of year to make aromatherapy recipes, because you can give them as Mother's Day gifts. Your mom will love to receive some of the items we have recipes for this month, including massage oils, skin care products, hair care products, and even a few items for around the home.

May 1

Aromatherapy Temptation Massage Oil

Materials

- ½ ounce rice bran oil
- 7 drops tea tree oil
- 5 drops peppermint essential oil
- 5 drops marjoram essential oil

Directions

Combine ingredients together in a glass bowl. To use massage into skin with fingertips.

May 2

Aromatherapy Erotic Massage Oil

Materials

- ½ ounce rice bran oil
- 10 drops jasmine essential oil
- 8 drops ylang ylang essential oil

Directions

Combine ingredients together in a glass bowl. To use massage into skin with fingertips.

May 3

Aromatherapy Anti-Cellulite Massage Oil

Materials

- ½ ounce rice bran oil
- 6 drops lavender essential oil
- 6 drops rosemary essential oil
- 6 drops juniper essential oil

Directions

Combine ingredients together in a glass bowl. To use massage into skin with fingertips.

May 4

Aromatherapy Perfumed Massage Oil

Materials

- ½ ounce rice bran oil
- 10 drops jasmine essential oil
- 10 drops lavender essential oil
- 5 drops rose essential oil

Directions

Combine ingredients together in a glass bowl. To use massage into skin with fingertips.

May 5

Cleansing Lotion

Materials

- ¼ C jojoba oil
- 7 drops bergamot essential oil
- 8 drops sweet orange essential oil
- 4 drops lavender essential oil

Directions

Combine ingredients together and store in a dark colored glass bottle. To use, apply a few drops to face and rub gently with your fingers. Rinse with clear, warm water.

May 6

Aromatherapy Toner for Oily Skin

Materials

- 1 C witch hazel
- 15 drops eucalyptus essential oil
- 5 drops geranium essential oil
- 5 drops peppermint essential oil
- 8 drops rosemary essential oil

Directions

Combine ingredients in a glass bowl and transfer to an airtight container. Shake well before each use.

May 7

Aromatherapy Cleansing Lotion

Materials

- ¼ C rice bran oil
- 8 drops lavender essential oil
- 6 drops geranium essential oil
- 5 drops rose essential oil

Directions

Combine ingredients in a glass bowl and transfer to an airtight container. Shake well before each use.

May 8

Aromatherapy Facial Mist for Skin Toning

Materials

- 4 ounces pure distilled water
- 12 drops lavender essential oil
- 8 drops bergamot essential oil
- 2 drops chamomile essential oil
- 2 drops rosewood essential oil

Directions

Combine ingredients together in a spray bottle. Shake well before each use.

May 9

Aromatherapy Skin Cleansing Lotion

Materials

- ¼ C jojoba oil
- 10 drops rose essential oil
- 5 drops jasmine essential oil
- 5 drops geranium essential oil
- 2 drops ylang ylang essential oil

Directions

Combine ingredients in a glass bowl and transfer them to a dark colored glass bottle. Shake well before each use.

May 10

Aromatherapy Moisturizing Cream

Materials

- ½ C rice bran oil
- 3 ounces rosewater
- ½ ounce grated beeswax
- 10 drops rose essential oil
- 5 drops lavender essential oil
- 5 drops sweet orange essential oil
- 6 drops palmarosa essential oil
- 6 drops sandalwood essential oil

Directions

In a double boiler over medium heat, combine the beeswax and rice bran oil. When ingredients have melted and blended together, remove from heat. Pour water into a bowl and start blending with an electric mixer. As the water is spinning, add the beeswax mixture. Blend until mixture is emulsified. Add the essential oils, and transfer mixture to covered containers.

May 11

Aromatic Body Lotion for Normal Skin

Materials

- ½ C unscented body lotion
- 12 drops lavender essential oil
- 6 drops rose essential oil
- 6 drops bergamot essential oil

Directions

Combine all ingredients together in a glass bowl. Transfer to covered containers.

May 12

Aromatic Body Lotion for Dry Skin

Materials

- ½ C unscented body lotion
- 8 drops lavender essential oil
- 8 drops geranium essential oil

- 8 drops rosewood essential oil

Directions

Combine all ingredients together in a glass bowl. Transfer to covered containers.

May 13

Aromatic Body Lotion for Oily Skin

Materials

- ½ C unscented body lotion
- 8 drops cypress essential oil
- 8 drops cedarwood essential oil
- 4 drops patchouli essential oil

Directions

Combine all ingredients together in a glass bowl. Transfer to covered containers.

May 14

Aromatic Body Lotion for Mature Skin

Materials

- ½ C unscented body lotion
- 8 drops frankincense essential oil
- 8 drops lavender essential oil
- 4 drops patchouli essential oil

Directions

Combine all ingredients together in a glass bowl. Transfer to covered containers.

May 15

Anti-Cellulite Skin Lotion

Materials

- ½ C unscented body lotion
- 1 ½ tbsp. witch hazel
- 24 drops lavender essential oil
- 20 drops juniper essential oil

- 20 drops geranium essential oil

Directions

Combine all ingredients together in a glass bowl. Transfer to covered containers.

May 16

Aromatherapy Minty Tooth Powder

Materials

- ½ C baking soda
- 1 tsp sea salt
- 35 drops peppermint essential oil
- 2 tsp myrrh powder

Directions

Combine all ingredients together and store in an airtight container. To use, dampen your toothbrush, and dip it into a teaspoon of the powder. Brush and rinse as normal.

May 17

Aromatherapy Minty Toothpaste

Materials

- ½ C baking soda
- 4 tbsp vegetable glycerin
- 10 drops peppermint essential oil
- 10 drops spearmint essential oil
- 5 drops cinnamon essential oil

Directions

Combine all ingredients together and store in an airtight container. Use just like regular toothpaste.

May 18

Aromatherapy Citrus Mint Mouthwash

Materials

- 1 C vodka
- 15 drops orange essential oil

- 15 drops peppermint essential oil
- 5 drops eucalyptus essential oil

Directions

Combine all ingredients together and store in an airtight bottle.

May 19

Aromatherapy Chest Congestion Rub

Materials

- 1 tbsp emu oil
- 12 drops eucalyptus essential oil

Directions

Combine ingredients together and rub on chest twice daily.

May 20

Aromatherapy Bath for Colds

Materials

- 12 drops eucalyptus essential oil

Directions

Add essential oil to bath water (under the running water for better distribution). Soak for at least 15 minutes.

May 21

Cold and Cough Diffuser Blend

Materials

- 8 drops eucalyptus essential oil
- 5 drops thyme essential oil
- 5 drops lemon essential oil
- 5 drops rosemary essential oil

Directions

Combine ingredients in your diffuser and use as instructed.

May 22

Anti-Anxiety Diffuser Blend 1

Materials

- 3 drops bergamot essential oil
- 2 drops lavender essential oil
- 1 drop frankincense essential oil

Directions

Combine ingredients in your diffuser and use as instructed.

May 23

Anti-Anxiety Diffuser Blend 2

Materials

- 3 drops bergamot essential oil
- 2 drops lavender essential oil
- 2 drops chamomile essential oil

Directions

Combine ingredients in your diffuser and use as instructed.

May 24

Aromatherapy Foot Treatment for High Blood Pressure

Materials

- 3 drops lavender essential oil
- 3 drops ylang ylang essential oil
- 3 drops marjoram essential oil

Directions

Mix oils in the palm of your hand and apply to the soles of your feet.

May 25

High Blood Pressure Diffuser Blend

Materials

- 15 drops clary sage essential oil
- 10 drops lavender essential oil
- 6 drops ylang ylang essential oil
- 4 drops marjoram essential oil

Directions

Combine all ingredients together in a glass bowl. Transfer to a covered, dark colored glass container. Add a few drops to the diffuser when needed.

May 26

Aromatherapy Bath for High Blood Pressure

Materials

- 4 drops ylang ylang essential oil
- 2 drops clary sage essential oil
- 1 drop marjoram essential oil

Directions

Combine oils in a glass bowl and add to bath water, under running water for better dispersion. Soak for at least 20 minutes.

May 27

Aromatherapy Shampoo for Hair Loss

Materials

- 1 C liquid Castile soap
- 90 drops laurel hydrosol
- 30 drops vegetable oil
- 20 drops hypericum essential oil
- 10 drops lavender essential oil
- 5 drops laurel essential oil
- 5 drops rosemary essential oil

Directions

Combine all ingredients together in a glass bowl. Transfer to an empty shampoo bottle. Use in place of your regular shampoo to combat hair loss.

May 28

Aromatic Insect Repellant

Materials

- 3 ½ tbsp. rice bran oil
- 5 drops eucalyptus essential oil
- 8 drops citronella essential oil
- 5 drops lavender essential oil
- 5 drops cedarwood essential oil
- 5 drops rosemary essential oil

Directions

Combine all ingredients together in a spray bottle. Use whenever you are outdoors.

May 29

Aromatic Moth Repellant

Materials

- 3 ½ tbsp. lavender carrier oil
- 25 drops cedarwood essential oil
- 20 drops bassilicum essential oil
- 15 drops eucalyptus essential oil
- 20 drops lemon essential oil
- 10 drops lavender essential oil
- 10 drops lemongrass essential oil

Directions

Combine all ingredients in a glass bowl. Transfer to a dark colored glass bottle. To use, soak cotton balls in mixture and place in drawers and closets to keep moths away.

May 30

Aromatherapy Candle for Frustration

Materials

- 1 C grated beeswax
- 1 cotton wick
- 1 small Mason jar
- 3 drops jasmine essential oil
- 3 drops chamomile essential oil

Directions

In a double boiler over medium heat, melt the beeswax. Remove from heat, add the essential oils. Pour ¼ of the mixture into the Mason jar, and add the wick. While holding the wick steady, add the rest of the wax mixture.

May 31

Aromatherapy Candle for Nerves

Materials

- 1 C grated beeswax
- 1 cotton wick
- 1 small Mason jar
- 3 drops jasmine essential oil
- 3 drops pathouli essential oil

Directions

In a double boiler over medium heat, melt the beeswax. Remove from heat, add the essential oils. Pour ¼ of the mixture into the Mason jar, and add the wick. While holding the wick steady, add the rest of the wax mixture.

White Lemon

The Benefits of Aromatherapy

Many people don't realize just how many benefits, both physical and mental, aromatherapy can offer. While a lot of people use it simply for relaxation, there are numerous other benefits. In fact, aromatherapy is so beneficial it would take an entire book to tell you about the benefits. So, for the sake of keeping things short for this e-book, we are going to discuss the top four benefits of aromatherapy.

1) **Stress Reduction** – One of the main reasons why people swear by aromatherapy is the fact that it is so helpful for stress reduction. Think about it. When was the last time you smelled home-baked bread and didn't feel happy and relaxed? Certain smells trigger certain emotions, and these scents can help to alleviate a lot of the stress in your life. Aromatherapy may not get rid of your stressors, but it will make it a whole lot easier to deal with them. In addition to reducing stress, aromatherapy can also help to alleviate pain that can cause a lot of your stress.
2) **Fighting Depression** – Aromatherapy is often recommended for those who are suffering from depression. Many of the scents are extremely uplifting, and will go a great distance to lift your spirits. A massage with essential oils is one of the best ways to deal with depression, and it also helps to get rid of the aches and pains of the day. Particular scents, such as citrus, are uplifting and often used to help those who suffer from depression.
3) **Pain Management** – As previously mentioned, aromatherapy is great for pain management. When the body is able to relax, it is a lot easier to deal with pain. One essential oil that is particularly good for pain relief is clary sage. It is really good for those who deal with menstrual pain.
4) **Blood Pressure Management** – Doctors often recommend aromatherapy for patients who have problem with high blood pressure or hypertension. The reason why it helps is because it is relaxing. When you are able to relax, your blood pressure will lower and be in a healthier range. Some of the best essential oils for managing blood pressure include lavender and rosemary, because they are so soothing.

June

Summer is here, and it is time to watch out for the harsh rays of the sun. Aromatherapy preparations can help with sun protection, as well as after-sun care. This month, you will find recipes for sunscreen and after-sun care, as well as other skin and hair care recipes. We also have a whole lot of awesome candle recipes for you, so you can enjoy aromatherapy at any time simply by lighting a candle.

June 1

Aromatherapy Lip Balm

Materials

- 3 tbsp grated beeswax
- 1 tsp rice bran oil
- 3 drops peppermint essential oil

Directions

In a double boiler over medium heat, melt the beeswax with the rice bran oil. When ingredients have melted and blended together, remove from heat and add the peppermint essential oil. Pour into a prepared lip balm tub or tube.

June 2

Aromatherapy Bath Salts

Materials

- 1 C Epsom salts
- 1 C coarse sea salt
- 10 drops lemon essential oil

Directions

Combine all ingredients together in a glass bowl. Transfer to an airtight container to store. To use, add ½ C of the mixture to your bath water.

June 3

Skin Refreshing Mud Mask

Materials

- 2 tbsp kaolin clay
- 1 tsp liquid aloe vera
- 2 drops lavender essential oil
- 3 drops rosemary essential oil
- 1 drop peppermint essential oil

Directions

Combine all ingredients together in a glass bowl. To use, apply all over face, avoiding your eyes. Let the mask sit for 10 minutes, then rinse with clear, warm water.

June 4

Spring Fresh Diffuser Blend

Materials

- 3 drops eucalyptus essential oil
- 2 drops pine essential oil
- 2 drops lemongrass essential oil

Directions

Combine ingredients in your diffuser and use as instructed.

June 5

Sunny Day Diffuser Blend

Materials

- 3 drops sweet orange essential oil
- 2 drops lemon essential oil
- 2 drops lemongrass essential oil

Directions

Combine ingredients in your diffuser and use as instructed.

June 6

Lemon Fresh Dish Liquid

Materials

- 2 C liquid Castile soap
- 15 drops lemon essential oil
- 5 drops sweet orange essential oil

Directions

Combine ingredients together and transfer to a clean dish liquid bottle. Use as you would regular dish liquid.

June 7

Aromatherapy Candle for Concentration

Materials

- 1 C grated beeswax
- 1 cotton wick
- 1 small Mason jar
- 5 drops lemon essential oil
- 5 drops jasmine essential oil

Directions

In a double boiler over medium heat, melt the beeswax. Remove from heat, add the essential oils. Pour ¼ of the mixture into the Mason jar, and add the wick. While holding the wick steady, add the rest of the wax mixture.

June 8

Aromatherapy Candle for Mourning

Materials

- 1 C grated beeswax
- 1 cotton wick
- 1 small Mason jar
- 4 drops clary sage essential oil
- 4 drops rosemary essential oil
- 3 drops marjoram essential oil

Directions

In a double boiler over medium heat, melt the beeswax. Remove from heat, add the essential oils. Pour ¼ of the mixture into the Mason jar, and add the wick. While holding the wick steady, add the rest of the wax mixture.

June 9

Aromatherapy Candle for Anxiety Relief

Materials

- 1 C grated beeswax
- 1 cotton wick
- 1 small Mason jar

- 10 drops lavender essential oil
- 5 drops rose geranium essential oil

Directions

In a double boiler over medium heat, melt the beeswax. Remove from heat, add the essential oils. Pour ¼ of the mixture into the Mason jar, and add the wick. While holding the wick steady, add the rest of the wax mixture.

June 10

Aromatherapy Morning After Candle

Materials

- 1 C grated beeswax
- 1 cotton wick
- 1 small Mason jar
- 5 drops jasmine essential oil
- 5 drops grapefruit essential oil
- 3 drops tangerine essential oil

Directions

In a double boiler over medium heat, melt the beeswax. Remove from heat, add the essential oils. Pour ¼ of the mixture into the Mason jar, and add the wick. While holding the wick steady, add the rest of the wax mixture.

June 11

Aromatherapy Candle for Cold Relief

Materials

- 1 C grated beeswax
- 1 cotton wick
- 1 small Mason jar
- 10 drops peppermint essential oil
- 5 drops eucalyptus essential oil

Directions

In a double boiler over medium heat, melt the beeswax. Remove from heat, add the essential oils. Pour ¼ of the mixture into the Mason jar, and add the wick. While holding the wick steady, add the rest of the wax mixture.

June 12

Aromatherapy Candle to Stay Awake

Materials

- 1 C grated beeswax
- 1 cotton wick
- 1 small Mason jar
- 8 drops cinnamon essential oil
- 5 drops clove essential oil
- 2 drops spiced apple essential oil

Directions

In a double boiler over medium heat, melt the beeswax. Remove from heat, add the essential oils. Pour ¼ of the mixture into the Mason jar, and add the wick. While holding the wick steady, add the rest of the wax mixture.

June 13

Aromatherapy Candle for Irritability

Materials

- 1 C grated beeswax
- 1 cotton wick
- 1 small Mason jar
- 10 drops rose essential oil
- 5 drops chamomile essential oil

Directions

In a double boiler over medium heat, melt the beeswax. Remove from heat, add the essential oils. Pour ¼ of the mixture into the Mason jar, and add the wick. While holding the wick steady, add the rest of the wax mixture.

June 14

Aromatherapy Candle for Romance

Materials

- 1 C grated beeswax
- 1 cotton wick
- 1 small Mason jar

- 8 drops jasmine essential oil
- 5 drops sandalwood essential oil
- 2 drops ylang ylang essential oil

Directions

In a double boiler over medium heat, melt the beeswax. Remove from heat, add the essential oils. Pour ¼ of the mixture into the Mason jar, and add the wick. While holding the wick steady, add the rest of the wax mixture.

June 15

Deep Breathing Diffuser Blend

Materials

- 1 drop bergamot essential oil
- 1 drop ylang ylang essential oil
- 1 drop patchouli essential oil

Directions

Combine ingredients in your diffuser and use as instructed.

June 16

Floral Diffuser Blend

Materials

- 2 drops geranium essential oil
- 2 drops rose essential oil
- 2 drops lavender essential oil

Directions

Combine ingredients in your diffuser and use as instructed.

June 17

Odor-Fighting Diffuser Blend

Materials

- 3 drops lemon essential oil

- 2 drops cilantro essential oil
- 1 drop lime essential oil

Directions

Combine ingredients in your diffuser and use as instructed.

June 18

Fresh-Scent Diffuser Blend

Materials

- 2 drops lavender essential oil
- 2 drops lemon essential oil
- 2 drops rosemary essential oil

Directions

Combine ingredients in your diffuser and use as instructed.

June 19

Aromatherapy Cuticle Treatment

Materials

- ½ ounce rice bran oil
- 5 drops tea tree oil

Directions

Combine ingredients together and transfer to a dark colored glass bottle. To use, apply to cuticles and massage gently.

June 20

Aromatherapy Body Powder

Materials

- 25 drops lavender essential oil
- 10 drops rose essential oil
- ½ C arrowroot powder

Directions

Combine ingredients together in a glass bowl. Transfer to an airtight container.

June 21

Aromatherapy Body Powder for Oily Skin

Materials
- ½ C kaolin clay powder
- 25 drops lavender essential oil
- 10 drops rose essential oil

Directions

Combine ingredients together in a glass bowl. Transfer to an airtight container.

June 22

Solid Perfume

Materials
- 1/8 ounce grated beeswax
- ½ ounce jojoba oil
- 4 drops lavender essential oil
- 3 drops ylang ylang essential oil

Directions

In a double boiler over medium heat, combine the beeswax and jojoba oil. When ingredients have melted and blended together, remove from heat. Add the essential oils and transfer mixture to a covered container.

June 23

Aromatic Shower Gel

Materials
- 1 C shower gel base
- 35 drops lavender essential oil
- 25 drops rose essential oil
- 10 drops geranium essential oil

Directions

Combine ingredients together in a glass bowl. Transfer to a covered container. Use just like regular shower gel.

June 24

Aromatherapy Linen Spray

Materials

- ½ C pure distilled water
- 20 drops chamomile essential oil
- 10 drops clary sage essential oil

Directions

Combine ingredients together in a spray bottle. Spritz betting as needed.

June 25

Aromatherapy Linen Spray 2

Materials

- ½ C pure distilled water
- 15 drops sandalwood essential oil
- 15 drops grapefruit essential oil
- 2 drops rose essential oil
- 2 drops jasmine essential oil

Directions

Combine ingredients together in a spray bottle. Spritz betting as needed.

June 26

Aromatherapy Dryer Sheets

Materials

- 5-5"X5" cotton fabric squares
- 5 drops lemon essential oil

Directions

Place 1 drop of essential oil per square of fabric. Use one square per laundry load. These are reusable, making them environmentally friendly.

June 27

Aromatherapy for Your Hair

Materials

- 1 drop rosemary essential oil
- Hair brush

Directions

Apply the rosemary essential oil to your hair brush, and brush hair as normal.

June 28

Shoe Deodorizer

Materials

- 4 tbsp baking soda
- 4 tbsp cornstarch
- 5 drops lavender essential oil

Directions

Combine baking soda and corn starch in a glass bowl. Slowly add the essential oil, stirring to mix. Store in an airtight container. To use, sprinkle mixture into shoes before bedtime so they smell fresh in the morning.

June 29

Aromatherapy Body Lotion

Materials

- 1 C unscented hand or body lotion
- 10 drops patchouli essential oil
- 20 drops sandalwood essential oil

Directions

Combine ingredients together in a glass bowl. Transfer to a lotion squeeze or pump bottle.

June 30

Aromatherapy Smelling Salts

Materials

- 4 tbsp coarse sea salt
- 30 drops lemon essential oil
- 10 drops peppermint essential oil
- Glass bowl

Directions

Combine ingredients together in the glass bowl. To use, hold the bowl a few inches from your nose and inhale deeply.

Aromatherapy and Children

The very first thing we need to tell you about essential oils and your kids is to keep ALL essential oils out of reach of your kids. These oils have very powerful healing properties, and therefore should be treated in the same manner as you would treat medications, household cleaners, and other things that could be poisonous to kids and pets. Essential oils are highly concentrated, and even a tiny drop could be extremely harmful to a child.

Lower the Dosage

Now, with that being said, essential oils are healthy for children when they are used properly. They should never be taken orally, unless your doctor has specifically advised you to do this. Otherwise, there is a risk of serious illness. When it comes to essential oils and kids, dosages should be much lower than they are for most of the recipes in this book. You will find plenty of recipes for children in this e-book, and the amounts have been adjusted so they are completely safe for kids to use. If you are using a steam inhalation method, make sure that your kids are always supervised, and that the inhalation is done for no longer than one minute.

Double the Dilution

Always make sure that you do not put undiluted essential oils on your kids' skin. Again, make sure that any blend you use for kids is half the strength of a regular blend. Basically, you will either want to cut the amount of essential oils you are using in a recipe in half, or double the amount of carrier oil you are using to make sure that the oils have the proper dilution. For instance, a skin lotion for adults may contain 10 drops of essential oils and one ounce of carrier oil. For children, the recipe would have five to six drops of essential oils and one ounce of carrier oil, or 10 drops of essential oils and two to three ounces of carrier oil.

Essential Oils for Kids

If you plan on using essential oil aromatherapy blends for your kids, it is a good idea to speak with your physician first to make sure that there won't be any health issues. This is especially important if your kids have any allergies. Your doctor can also recommend essential oils to use for certain health problems. Commonly used essential oils for mixtures for kids include lavender, chamomile, and tea tree oil. There are many essential oils that you should never use in preparations for children, as they are just too strong. These include:

- Clove
- Basil
- Black pepper
- Peppermint
- Patchouli
- Lemon verbena

If you do plan on using essential oils in treatments for children, you should invest in a good book about the various essential oils and how they are used. The more you know, the healthier your family is going to be.

July

Summer is here, and it is important that you take care of your skin. It is also a time when you can easily catch that dreaded summer cold. So, with these things in mind, we are offering up some great aromatherapy skin care recipes, cold and flu preparations, and more. Enjoy a variety of diffuser blends, as well as recipes for bath products that will help keep your skin smooth and silky.

July 1

Romantic Diffuser Blend

Materials

- 3 drops ylang ylang essential oil
- 2 drops sandalwood essential oil
- 1 drop rosemary essential oil

Directions

Combine ingredients in your diffuser and use as instructed.

July 2

Diffuser Blend for Hangovers

Materials

- 2 drops cinnamon essential oil
- 2 drops ginger essential oil
- 2 drops clove essential oil
- 1 drop sandalwood essential oil

Directions

Combine ingredients in your diffuser and use as instructed.

July 3

Confidence Boosting Diffuser Blend

Materials

- 4 drops lemon essential oil
- 3 drops rosemary essential oil
- 1 drop basil essential oil

Directions

Combine ingredients in your diffuser and use as instructed.

July 4

Sleepy Time Diffuser Blend

Materials

- 2 drops sandalwood essential oil
- 2 drops juniper essential oil
- 1 drop ylang ylang essential oil

Directions

Combine ingredients in your diffuser and use as instructed.

July 5

Revitalizing Diffuser Blend

Materials

- 3 drops peppermint essential oil
- 2 drops lemon essential oil
- 1 drop lime essential oil

Directions

Combine ingredients in your diffuser and use as instructed.

July 6

Germ Fighting Diffuser Blend

Materials

- 2 drops tea tree oil
- 2 drops neroli essential oil
- 2 drops eucalyptus essential oil
- 1 drop thyme essential oil

Directions

Combine ingredients in your diffuser and use as instructed.

July 7

Headache Relieving Diffuser Blend

Materials

- 4 drops lavender essential oil
- 3 drops peppermint essential oil
- 1 drop rose essential oil

Directions

Combine ingredients in your diffuser and use as instructed.

July 8

Stress Relief Diffuser Blend

Materials

- 3 drops clary sage essential oil
- 2 drops lemon essential oil
- 1 drop lavender essential oil

Directions

Combine ingredients in your diffuser and use as instructed.

July 9

Massage Oil for Sore Joints

Materials

- 1 C jojoba oil
- 16 drops eucalyptus essential oil
- 16 drops cinnamon essential oil
- 15 drops sweet orange essential oil
- 6 drops vitamin E oil
- 1 tsp liquid aloe vera

Directions

Combine all ingredients together in a glass bowl. Transfer mixture to a dark colored glass bottle. To use, apply to affected areas and massage gently with your fingertips.

July 10

Energizing Bath Blend

Materials

- 4 ounces rice bran oil
- 10 drops lemon essential oil
- 4 drops eucalyptus essential oil
- 2 drops cinnamon essential oil

Directions

Combine all ingredients together in a glass bowl. Transfer to a dark colored glass bottle. To use, add 2 tsp of the mixture to your bath water.

July 11

Energizing Foot Bath

Materials

- 2 ounces jojoba oil
- 5 drops lemon essential oil
- 1 drop cinnamon essential oil
- 1 drop peppermint essential oil

Directions

Combine all ingredients together in a glass bowl. Transfer to a dark colored glass bottle. To use, add 1 tsp of the mixture to your foot soak basin.

July 12

Sweet Smelling Sachet

Materials

- 10 drops rose essential oil
- 5 drops lavender essential oil
- 3 drops chamomile essential oil
- Foam makeup sponges
- Sachet bags

365 Days of Aromatherapy

Directions

Combine essential oils together in a glass bowl. Place a few drops of the mixture onto each sponge. Place 1-2 sponges in each sachet bag.

July 13

Scented Mineral Bath

Materials

- 2 tbsp sea salt
- 1 tbsp baking soda
- 1 ½ tsp borax powder
- 6 drops lemon essential oil
- 3 drops ylang ylang essential oil

Directions

Combine all ingredients together in a glass bowl. Pour mixture under running bathwater to make sure that the salt dissolves and mixture mixes into the water.

July 14

Aromatherapy Play Dough

Materials

- ½ C corn starch
- ½ C brown rice flour
- ½ C salt
- 1 tsp cream of tartar
- ½ C water
- ½ tsp essential oils of choice
- 1 tsp food grade colorant of choice

Directions

In a double boiler over medium heat, combine rice flour, salt, cream of tartar, and food coloring. Stir until mixture forms a ball and remove from heat. Add essential oils and knead well to distribute scent evenly. Store in an airtight container when not in use.

July 15

Relaxation Massage Oil

Directions

- 1 ounce rice bran oil
- 3 drops lavender essential oil
- 3 drops tangerine essential oil
- 3 drops marjoram essential oil
- 1 drop chamomile essential oil

Directions

Combine all ingredients together in a glass bowl. Transfer mixture to a dark colored glass bottle. To use, apply a few drops to tired, achy joints and massage gently with your fingertips.

July 16

Aromatherapy Bath

Materials

- 3 drops lemon essential oil
- 3 drops peppermint essential oil

Directions

Add essential oils directly under running bathwater. Soak for at least 20 minutes.

July 17

Stinky Dog Spray

Materials

- 1 ounce pure distilled water
- 8 drops lavender essential oil
- 8 drops geranium essential oil
- 5 drops lemon essential oil

Directions

Combine all ingredients together in a spray bottle. To use, shake well, hold at least 10" from dog, and spray onto coat, avoiding the eyes.

July 18

Bath Goo

Materials

- ½ C aloe vera gel
- ½ C raw honey
- ½ C coarse sea salt
- ½ C heavy cream
- 10 drops lemon essential oil

Directions

Combine ingredients together in a glass bowl. Transfer mixture to an airtight container, and use half in your bath water. Store the remainder of the mixture in the fridge for up to one week.

July 19

Refreshing Skin Mist

Materials

- 10 ounces pure distilled water
- 2 tsp extra virgin olive oil
- 10 drops rosemary essential oil
- 2 drops lavender essential oil

Directions

Combine all ingredients together in a spray bottle. To use, mist on skin when skin is still moist after getting out of the tub or shower.

July 20

Cold and Flu Inhaler

Materials

- 1 tbsp extra virgin olive oil
- 10 drops tea tree oil
- Tissues

Directions

Combine olive oil and tea tree oil together in a dark colored glass bottle. To use, place a couple of drops on a tissue and inhale.

July 21

Congestion Inhaler

Materials

- 1 tbsp extra virgin olive oil
- 3 drops lavender essential oil
- 2 drops rosemary essential oil
- 2 drops tea tree oil
- Tissues

Directions

Combine olive oil and essential oils together in a dark colored glass bottle. To use, place a couple of drops on a tissue and inhale.

July 22

Headache Rub

Materials

- 1 tbsp rice bran oil
- 5 drops lavender essential oil
- 1 drop peppermint essential oil

Directions

Combine ingredients together in a glass bowl. Transfer mixture to a dark colored glass bottle. To use, apply a couple of drops to your temples and massage gently with your fingertips.

July 23

Muscle Pain Rub

Materials

- 2 tbsp rice bran oil
- 5 drops lavender essential oil
- 5 drops chamomile essential oil

Directions

Combine ingredients together in a glass bowl. Transfer mixture to a dark colored glass bottle. To use, apply a couple of drops to affected areas and massage gently with your fingertips.

July 24

Sweet Orange Chocolates

Materials

- 1 box of chocolates
- Absorbent paper
- 5-6 drops sweet orange essential oil

Directions

Apply the sweet orange essential oil to the absorbent paper with an eye dropper. Place paper inside the box of chocolates. Set in a dark place for 24-48 hours. The chocolate will absorb the scent and flavor of the essential oil.

July 25

Cellulite Blend

Materials

- 3 ounces hazelnut oil
- 2 drops eucalyptus essential oil
- 2 drops lemon essential oil
- 2 drops cedarwood essential oil
- 2 drops sage essential oil
- 2 drops cypress essential oil
- 2 drops niaouli essential oil

Directions

Combine all ingredients together in a glass bowl. Transfer mixture to a dark colored glass bottle. To use, apply a couple of drops onto affected areas and massage gently with your fingertips, twice daily.

July 26

Aromatherapy Bookmark

Materials

- 1 bookmark
- 2 drops sweet orange essential oil
- 1 drop grapefruit essential oil

Directions

Combine essential oils, and place them on the bookmark with an eye dropper. Let sit in a dark place to dry.

July 27

Peppermint Bath Salts

Materials

- 1 C Epsom salts
- 1 C coarse sea salt
- 5 drops peppermint essential oil

Directions

Combine all ingredients together in a glass bowl. Transfer mixture to an airtight container. To use, add ½ C of the mixture to your bathwater.

July 28

Menstrual Cramp Relief Bath Salts

Materials

- ¼ C Epsom salts
- ¼ C coarse sea salt
- 5 drops lavender essential oil
- 2 drops cypress essential oil
- 2 drops nutmeg essential oil
- 2 drops peppermint essential oil

Directions

Combine all ingredients together in a glass bowl and add mixture to your bathwater. Soak for at least 20 minutes.

July 29

Aromatherapy Skin Toner

Materials

- 2 ounces steeped green tea, chilled
- 5 drops lavender essential oil

- 5 drops geranium essential oil

Directions

Combine all ingredients together in a dark colored glass bottle. To use, shake well, apply a few drops of the mixture to a cotton pad, and apply to face and neck after cleansing.

July 30

Aromatherapy Bath Melts

Materials

- ½ C cocoa butter
- ½ C baking soda
- ¼ C citric acid
- Powdered herbs of choice

Directions

In a double boiler over medium heat, melt the cocoa butter. Remove from heat and add the powdered ingredients. Pour mixture into prepared molds and allow to set for 24-48 hours.

July 31

Aromatherapy Bath Fizzies

Materials

- 1 C baking soda
- ½ C corn starch
- ½ C citric acid
- 10 drops lemon essential oil
- 5 drops sweet orange essential oil
- Food grade colorant (optional)

Directions

Combine all ingredients together in a glass bowl. Press mixture into prepared molds, and allow to set for 24-48 hours before using.

Types of Aromatherapy Diffusers

When it comes to aromatherapy via diffusers, you may be confused, because there are so many different types of diffusers out there. Basically, they all have the same final outcome: the scent is delivered so you can breathe it in. But, there are different ways that the diffusers use to deliver the scents. Let's take a look at the various types of diffusers that are available.

- Nebulizer – This is just like a regular nebulizer. It allows essential oils to be dispersed as molecules so they spread better. This method is often used for pain and anxiety relief.
- Electric Oil Diffuser – This type of diffuser lets you mix any scent you like and then send the scent throughout your home. Choose from spa scent diffusers, scent balls, car fresheners, and fan diffusers.
- Oil Diffuser – There are two types of oil diffusers that are safe to use around children and pets: night lights and jewelry. Both release small amounts of scent.
- Oil Burner – This is great for beginners in aromatherapy. The oil is heated on a platform that rests just above the heat source, such as a candle. You do need to be careful with this type of diffuser, as it is a fire risk.
- Air Freshener – This is such an easy way to enjoy aromatherapy. All you have to do is add a few drops to an ounce of pure distilled water, and spray around your home.
- Candles – Candles are growing in popularity all the time, particularly aromatherapy candles. You can find them in just about any scent imaginable, and we have included recipes in this e-book so you can make your own aromatherapy candles.
- Diffuser for Skin Care – You can use several types of diffusers for skin care. One of the best types is one that operates on steam. Or, you can make you own steam diffuser with a bowl, a towel, boiling water, and essential oils.
- USB Aromatherapy – Enjoy using this portable aromatherapy diffuser that you can take anywhere. All you need is a computer or another device with a USB port to plug it into. Add a drop of your favorite essential oil, and it is all ready to go.
- Car Diffuser – If you want to keep your car smelling fresh, you need a car aromatherapy diffuser. It can be plugged into what used to be the cigarette lighter (now a port for plugging in electrical items). This is a great idea for those who smoke in their vehicles.
- Inhaler – A nasal inhaler is a great way to get the full effects of aromatherapy. It is small and easy to carry around in a purse or in your pocket, and you can use your favorite scents whenever you need a pick-me-up.

August

Summer is winding down, but there are still a lot more warm days to enjoy before fall arrives. This means that you need to protect your skin from the summer sun, and be vigilant about after-sun care. So, that is why we have all kinds of great aromatherapy recipes for your skin this month. There are also recipes for sweet-smelling body sprays, and of course plenty of diffuser and other recipes.

August 1

Vaginal Dryness Blend

Materials

- ¾ C jojoba oil
- ¼ C melted cocoa butter
- 3 drops sandalwood essential oil
- 1 drop geranium essential oil

Directions

Combine ingredients together in a glass bowl while the coconut oil is still warm (melt in a double boiler over medium heat to keep from burning it). When mixture solidifies, transfer it to an airtight container. To use, apply a bit of the mixture to the vaginal area twice daily, and prior to intercourse.

August 2

Aromatherapy Foot Powder

Materials

- 1 C corn starch
- 1 tbsp baking soda
- 15 drops peppermint essential oil
- 5 drops tea tree oil

Directions

Combine all ingredients together in a glass bowl. Transfer mixture to an airtight container. To use, sprinkle on feet as needed.

August 3

Morning Body Scrub

Materials

- ½ C coarse sea salt
- ½ C corn meal
- 2/3 C rice bran oil
- 4 drops ginger essential oil
- 8 drops peppermint essential oil
- 6 drops rosemary essential oil

Directions

Combine all ingredients together in a glass bowl. Transfer mixture to an airtight container. Use as you would any body scrub..

August 4

Aromatherapy Body Spritzer

Materials

- ½ C pure distilled water
- 25 drops chamomile essential oil
- 10 drops lavender essential oil
- 5 drops rose essential oil

Directions

Combine all ingredients together in a spray bottle. Shake well before each use.

August 5

Aromatherapy Citrus Body Spray

Materials

- 1 C pure distilled water
- 10 drops lemon essential oil
- 10 drops lime essential oil
- 10 drops grapefruit essential oil
- 10 drops sweet orange essential oil
- 10 drops tangerine essential oil
- 5 drops lemongrass essential oil

Directions

Combine all ingredients together in a spray bottle. Shake well before each use.

August 6

Aromatherapy Hot Rock Massage

Materials

- Large, flat, smooth stones

- 1 ounce rice bran oil
- 10 drops chamomile essential oil
- 5 drops rose essential oil

Directions

Combine rice bran oil and essential oils in a dark colored glass bottle. To use, warm stones in the oven (warm, not hot), and rub some of the essential oil mixture onto each stone. Use stones as you would with a regular hot rock massage.

August 7

Peaceful Massage Oil

Directions

- 1 ounce rice bran oil
- 3 drops patchouli essential oil
- 3 drops sandalwood essential oil

Directions

Combine all ingredients together in a dark colored glass bottle. To use, apply a couple of drops of the mixture into the skin and gently massage.

August 8

Citrus Bath Salts

Materials

- 1 C Epsom salts
- 1 C coarse sea salt
- 1 C baking soda
- 12 drops lemon essential oil
- 6 drops lemongrass essential oil
- 6 drops sweet orange essential oil

Directions

Combine all ingredients together in a glass bowl. Transfer mixture to an airtight container. To use, add ½ C of the mixture to your bathwater.

August 9

Aromatherapy Disinfecting Spray

Materials

- ½ C pure distilled water
- 25 drops tea tree oil
- 12 drops eucalyptus essential oil
- 12 drops lemon essential oil

Directions

Combine all ingredients together in a spray bottle. Shake well before each use.

August 10

Aromatherapy Cold and Flu Steam

Materials

- 4 drops pine essential oil
- 4 drops eucalyptus essential oil
- 3 drops lemon essential oil

Directions

Fill a glass bowl with boiling water. Add the essential oils, and lean over the bowl, covering your head and the bowl with a towel. Inhale the vapors for up to 5 minutes.

August 11

Aromatherapy Aphrodisiac Bath Blend

Materials

- 4 tbsp heavy cream
- 3 drops Turkish rose-otto essential oil
- 2 drops jasmine essential oil

Directions

Combine all ingredients together in a glass bowl. Pour mixture into bathwater and soak for 20 minutes.

August 12

Aromatherapy Beeswax Heart Ornaments

Materials

- 1 pound grated beeswax
- 5-6 drops sweet orange essential oil
- Ribbon

Directions

In a double boiler over medium heat, melt the beeswax. Remove from heat, and add the sweet orange essential oil. Pour into heart shaped molds. When set, bore a hole through the top and run ribbon through for hanging.

August 13

Aromatherapy Honey Bath

Materials

- ¼ C raw honey
- 5 drops lavender essential oil
- 2 drops rose essential oil

Directions

Combine all ingredients together in a glass bowl. Transfer mixture to a dark colored glass bottle. To use, add a tablespoon or so of the mixture to your bathwater.

August 14

Vanilla Bath Fizzies

Materials

- 1 C baking soda
- ½ C corn starch
- ½ C citric acid
- 1 tsp melted cocoa butter
- 1 tsp vanilla essential oil

Directions

In a double boiler over medium heat, melt the coconut oil. Remove from heat, and add to dry ingredients. Add the essential oil. Pack mixture into molds and allow to dry for 24-48 hours.

August 15

Aromatherapy Ice Candles

Materials

- 1 pound paraffin wax
- 6 drops peppermint essential oil
- Glitter
- Cardboard milk carton
- Crushed ice
- Cotton wick

Directions

In a double boiler over medium heat, melt the paraffin wax. Remove from heat and add the peppermint essential oil and glitter. Cut the top section of the milk carton, and fill the carton with crushed ice, around a wick (the ice will hold the wick in place). Pour the wax mixture over the ice. Allow the mixture to cool, and peel away the carton. You will be left with a gorgeous candle that sparkles like ice.

August 16

Citrus Cuticle Soak

Materials

- 1 C pure distilled water
- 1 tbsp aloe vera gel
- 10 drops lemon essential oil

Directions

Combine all ingredients in a small glass bowl. To use, soak fingertips in the mixture for about 10 minutes.

August 17

Aromatherapy Glass and Surface Cleaner

Materials

- 1 C white vinegar
- 1 C pure distilled water
- ¼ C rubbing alcohol
- 10 drops rosemary essential oil
- 10 drops lemon essential oil
- 6 drops peppermint essential oil

Directions

Combine all ingredients together in a spray bottle. Shake well before each use.

August 18

Orange Glass Cleaner

Materials

- 1 C pure distilled water
- 1 C apple cider vinegar
- 2 tbsp Borax
- 2 tbsp orange essential oil
- 2 tbsp lemon essential oil

Directions

Combine all ingredients together in a spray bottle. Shake well before each use.

August 19

Aromatherapy Dish Liquid

Materials

- 1 C Castile liquid soap
- 10 drops lemon essential oil
- 10 drops orange essential oil

Directions

Combine all ingredients together in a squeeze bottle, and use as you would regular dish liquid.

August 20

Citrus Diffuser Blend

Materials

- 5 drops lime essential oil
- 3 drops sweet orange essential oil
- 1 drop cinnamon essential oil

Directions

Combine ingredients in your diffuser and use as instructed.

August 21

Perfumed Diffuser Blend

Materials

- 10 drops patchouli essential oil
- 6 drops vanilla essential oil
- 3 drops linden blossom essential oil
- 1 drop neroli essential oil

Directions

Combine ingredients in your diffuser and use as instructed.

August 22

Exotic Diffuser Blend

Materials

- 4 drops bergamot essential oil
- 3 drops sandalwood essential oil
- 3 drops grapefruit essential oil
- 1 drop jasmine essential oil

Directions

Combine ingredients in your diffuser and use as instructed.

August 23

Tranquil Diffuser Blend

Materials

- 4 drops bergamot essential oil
- 2 drops grapefruit essential oil
- 2 drops lemon essential oil
- 2 drops ylang ylang essential oil

Directions

Combine ingredients in your diffuser and use as instructed.

August 24

Aromatherapy Roll-On for Depression

Materials

- 24 drops bergamot essential oil
- 10 drops geranium essential oil
- 5 drops jasmine essential oil
- 15 drops lavender essential oil
- 3 drops cinnamon essential oil
- 3 drops rose essential oil
- Unscented roll-on

Directions

Add all of the essential oils to the unscented roll-on. To use, rub on neck, wrists, and chest as needed.

August 25

Anti-Bacterial Gel

Materials

- ½ C aloe vera gel
- 10 drops tea tree oil
- 3 drops orange essential oil
- 3 drops lime essential oil

Directions

Combine all ingredients together in a glass bowl. Transfer mixture to a small squeeze bottle. Use as you would regular anti-bacterial gel.

August 26

Appetite Suppressing Diffuser Blend

Materials

- 40 drops mandarin essential oil

- 12 drops peppermint essential oil
- 12 drops ginger essential oil
- 20 drops lemon essential oil

Directions

Combine all ingredients together and store in a dark colored glass bottle. To use, add a couple of drops of the mixture to the diffuser and use as instructed.

August 27

Diaper Rash Treatment

Materials

- 3 ounces jojoba oil
- 5 drops Roman chamomile essential oil
- 5 drops lavender essential oil

Directions

Combine all ingredients together in a glass bowl. Transfer mixture to a dark colored glass bottle. Shake well before each use.

August 28

Anti-Snoring Aromatherapy Roll-On

Materials

- 1 bottle of scent-free roll-on
- 8 drops lavender essential oil
- 8 drops geranium essential oil
- 8 drops marjoram essential oil
- 5 drops cedarwood essential oil
- 1 drop eucalyptus essential oil
- 1 drop frankincense essential oil

Directions

Add all of the essential oils to the roll-on. Apply to the chest, neck, and temples before going to bed.

August 29

Exfoliating Sugar Scrub

Materials

- 1 C sugar
- 1 ounce cold-pressed vegetable oil
- 1 ounce vegetable glycerin
- 1 ounce liquid Castile soap
- 3 drops vitamin E oil (liquid from 1 capsule)
- 8 drops peppermint essential oil

Directions

Combine all ingredients together in a glass bowl. Transfer mixture to an airtight container. Use as you would any exfoliating sugar scrub.

August 30

Whipped Body Butter

Materials

- 1 C shea butter
- 1 tbsp jojoba oil
- ½ tsp vitamin E oil
- 5 drops lemon essential oil

Directions

In a double boiler over medium heat, combine the shea butter, jojoba oil, and vitamin E oil. When ingredients have melted and blended together, remove from heat and add the lemon essential oil. Use an electric mixer or a whisk to whip the mixture until it is thick and creamy. Transfer mixture to a covered glass container.

August 31

Eucalyptus Oil

Materials

- 1 ounce rice bran oil
- 20 drops eucalyptus essential oil
- 10 drops lavender essential oil

Directions

Combine ingredients together in a dark colored glass bottle. Use for muscle, joint, and nerve pain by applying a few drops to the affected area and massaging gently before and after a warm bath.

White Lemon

Aromatherapy Essential Oil Must-Have's

Whether you plan on really getting into aromatherapy recipes, or you just want to use them when you need them, there are certain essential oils that no home should ever be without. These essential oils are loaded with healing properties, and can be used to make everything from skin creams to cold remedies and a whole lot more. Let's take a look at the five essential oils that you should always have in your home.

- Lavender – First of all, this oil has a beautiful, floral scent. It is also probably the most versatile of all of the essential oils. It can be used to treat anxiety and tension, and it can also be used to treat physical ailments, including burns, insect bites, and muscle pain. If you are looking for a scent to use for relaxing blends, lavender should be high on the list.
- Peppermint – Again, peppermint smells great, and it is loaded with medicinal properties. It is commonly used to treat stomach issues, and also for treating congestion. Peppermint is basically great for whatever ails you, from headaches to migraines to sore muscles to digestive issues, and a whole lot more.
- Eucalyptus – This is another go-to essential oil for colds, coughs, asthma, congestion, and more. It can also be used to treat wounds, and is often used in skin care products. You will find many recipes in this e-book that use eucalyptus, and you can also use it by itself in your bath or a diffuser.
- Lemon – Here is a fresh scent that can brighten any mood, and it can also help you concentrate and increase your awareness. Lemon is used in a lot of recipes in this e-book. It is used for household cleaning products, diffusers, skin care, bath products, perfumes, and more.
- Tea Tree Oil – When it comes to treating fungal infections, tea tree oil is definitely a must-have essential oil. It has been used in alternative medicine for centuries, and it has many uses. It is often recommended for treating toenail fungus and athlete's foot, and it can also help to heal minor wounds. It is also great for your hair, so try adding a few drops to your regular shampoo.

When you are buying essential oils, it is important to ensure that what you are getting is therapeutic grade, and 100 percent pure. You can find all of the essential oils you need for every recipe in this e-book at health food stores, and there are many online stores that offer complete catalogs of aromatherapy supplies.

September

The kids are back in school, leaving you with more time to play around with aromatherapy recipes. Because the kids are in school and picking up every germ that the other kids are passing around, it is a good idea to make some anti-bacterial products. This month, we have some great hand sanitizer recipes, as well as other anti-bacterial recipes that will keep colds, flus, and other illnesses away from your home.

September 1

Anti-Bacterial Blend

Materials

- 20 drops clove essential oil
- 20 drops lemon essential oil
- 12 drops cinnamon bark essential oil
- 10 drops eucalyptus essential oil
- 5 drops rosemary essential oil

Directions

Combine all ingredients together in a dark colored glass bottle. Store in a dark place, and use in other aromatherapy recipes. Shake well before each use.

September 2

Anti-Bacterial Hand Gel

Materials

- ½ C unscented aloe vera gel
- ½ ounce rubbing alcohol
- 10 drops Anti-Bacterial Blend

Directions

Combine all ingredients together in a glass bowl. Transfer mixture to a squeeze bottle and use just like a regular anti-bacterial hand gel.

September 3

Anti-Bacterial Shampoo

Materials

- 1 C liquid Castile soap
- 15 drops Anti-Bacterial Blend

Directions

Combine ingredients together in a glass bowl. Transfer mixture to an empty shampoo bottle.

September 4

Anti-Bacterial Hand Soap

Materials

- 1 pound clear glycerin melt and pour soap base
- 25 drops Anti-Bacterial Blend
- Food grade colorant (optional)

Directions

In a double boiler over medium heat, melt the glycerin soap base. Remove from heat and add the Anti-Bacterial Blend. Pour into soap molds and allow to set.

September 5

Anti-Bacterial Diffuser Blend

Materials

- 6 drops Anti-Bacterial Blend

Directions

Add Anti-Bacterial Blend to diffuser and use as instructed.

September 6

Anti-Bacterial Dish Liquid

Materials

- 2 C liquid Castile soap
- 25 drops Anti-Bacterial Blend

Directions

Combine ingredients together in a glass bowl. Transfer to a clean dish liquid bottle.

September 7

Insomnia Diffuser Blend

Materials

- 10 drops Roman chamomile essential oil
- 6 drops clary sage essential oil
- 5 drops bergamot essential oil

Directions

Combine ingredients in your diffuser and use as instructed.

September 8

Aromatherapy Room Mist 1

Materials

- ½ C pure distilled water
- 40 drops lime essential oil
- 30 drops bergamot essential oil
- 5 drops ylang ylang essential oil
- 2 drops rose essential oil

Directions

Combine ingredients together in a spray bottle. Shake well before each use.

September 9

Aromatherapy Room Mist 2

Materials

- ½ C pure distilled water
- 30 drops clary sage essential oil
- 10 drops lemon essential oil
- 5 drops lavender essential oil

Directions

Combine ingredients together in a spray bottle. Shake well before each use.

September 10

Aromatherapy Room Mist 3

Materials

- ½ C pure distilled water
- 40 drops rosemary essential oil
- 15 drops grapefruit essential oil
- 10 drops peppermint essential oil
- 3 drops spearmint essential oil

Directions

Combine ingredients together in a spray bottle. Shake well before each use.

September 11

Aromatherapy Room Mist 4

Materials

- ½ C pure distilled water
- 35 drops bergamot essential oil
- 30 drops spearmint essential oil

Directions

Combine ingredients together in a spray bottle. Shake well before each use.

September 12

Anxiety Diffuser Blend 1

Materials

- 2 drops bergamot essential oil
- 2 drops clary sage essential oil
- 1 drop frankincense essential oil

Directions

Combine ingredients in your diffuser and use as instructed.

September 13

Anxiety Diffuser Blend 2

Materials

- 3 drops sandalwood essential oil
- 3 drops bergamot essential oil

Directions

Combine ingredients in your diffuser and use as instructed.

September 14

Anxiety Diffuser Blend 3

Materials

- 3 drops lavender essential oil
- 3 drops clary sage essential oil

Directions

Combine ingredients in your diffuser and use as instructed.

September 15

Anxiety Diffuser Blend 4

Materials

- 2 drops mandarin orange essential oil
- 1 drop rose essential oil
- 1 drop lavender essential oil

Directions

Combine ingredients in your diffuser and use as instructed.

September 16

Aromatherapy Sugar Cube Scrub

Materials

- 11 ounces melt and pour soap base
- 2 C white sugar
- ½ C jojoba oil
- Liquid from a vitamin E capsule
- 4-5 drops pink grapefruit essential oil
- Pink food grade colorant (optional)

Directions

In a double boiler over medium heat, melt the soap base. Pour soap into a glass mixing bowl. Add vitamin E oil and jojoba oil, stirring to mix. While stirring, add the sugar and essential oils. At this point, the mixture will be thick and you can knead it with your hands. If using colorant, add it now. Pack mixture tightly into cube molds, and allow to dry for a couple of hours. If you don't have a cube mold, use a regular soap mold and cut the hardened bars into cubes.

September 17

Aromatherapy Insect Repellant

Materials

- ½ C pure distilled water
- 20 drops citronella essential oil
- 15 drops lavender essential oil
- 15 drops eucalyptus essential oil
- 10 drops lemongrass essential oil

Directions

Combine all ingredients together in a spray bottle. Shake well before each use.

September 18

Aromatherapy Facial Toner

Materials

- ¼ C witch hazel
- 1 ounce vodka
- 8 drops grapefruit essential oil

365 Days of Aromatherapy

- 5 drops cypress essential oil
- 3 drops tea tree oil

Directions

Combine all ingredients together in a glass bowl. Transfer to a dark colored glass bottle. To use, soak a makeup remover pad in solution and apply to face.

September 19

Aromatherapy Hair Conditioner

Materials

- 1 tbsp jojoba oil
- 3 drops rosemary essential oil

Directions

Combine ingredients together in a small glass bowl. To use, soak hair with warm water and apply mixture. Let the mixture sit on your hair for at least 15 minutes, rinse, and wash your hair as normal.

September 20

Simple Aromatherapy Perfume 1

Materials

- 1 tbsp jojoba oil
- 9 drops sandalwood essential oil
- 3 drops jasmine essential oil

Directions

Combine ingredients together in a glass bowl. Transfer mixture to a dark colored glass bottle. To use, apply a drop to each pulse point.

September 21

Simple Aromatherapy Perfume 2

Materials

- 1 tbsp jojoba oil
- 10 drops lemon essential oil

- 5 drops sweet orange essential oil
- 2 drops grapefruit essential oil
- 2 drops tangerine essential oil

Directions

Combine ingredients together in a glass bowl. Transfer mixture to a dark colored glass bottle. To use, apply a drop to each pulse point.

September 22

Simple Aromatherapy Perfume 3

Materials

- 1 tbsp jojoba oil
- 8 drops peppermint essential oil
- 8 drops lemon essential oil
- 5 drops lavender essential oil

Directions

Combine ingredients together in a glass bowl. Transfer mixture to a dark colored glass bottle. To use, apply a drop to each pulse point.

September 23

Simple Aromatherapy Perfume 4

Materials

- 1 tbsp jojoba oil
- 10 drops frankincense essential oil
- 5 drops rose essential oil
- 5 drops geranium essential oil
- 2 drops jasmine essential oil

Directions

Combine ingredients together in a glass bowl. Transfer mixture to a dark colored glass bottle. To use, apply a drop to each pulse point.

September 24

Simple Aromatherapy Perfume 5

Materials

- 1 tbsp jojoba oil
- 8 drops chamomile essential oil
- 5 drops rose essential oil
- 5 drops lavender essential oil
- 3 drops geranium essential oil
- 2 drops lemongrass essential oil

Directions

Combine ingredients together in a glass bowl. Transfer mixture to a dark colored glass bottle. To use, apply a drop to each pulse point.

September 25

Stretch Mark Blend

Materials

- ½ C cocoa butter
- 1 ounce rice bran oil
- 5 drops neroli essential oil

Directions

In a double boiler over medium heat, combine the cocoa butter and rice bran oil. When ingredients have melted and blended together, remove from heat and add the neroli essential oil. Pour mixture into a glass jar and allow to cool before using. To use, apply to affected areas and massage gently with your fingertips.

September 26

Stress Relieving Diffuser Blend 1

Materials

- 3 drops clary sage essential oil
- 2 drops lemon essential oil
- 1 drop lavender essential oil

Directions

Combine ingredients in your diffuser and use as instructed.

September 27

Stress Relieving Diffuser Blend 2

Materials

- 3 drops Roman chamomile essential oil
- 2 drops lavender essential oil
- 1 drop vetiver essential oil

Directions

Combine ingredients in your diffuser and use as instructed.

September 28

Stress Relieving Diffuser Blend 3

Materials

- 3 drops bergamot essential oil
- 2 drops geranium essential oil
- 1 drop frankincense essential oil

Directions

Combine ingredients in your diffuser and use as instructed.

September 29

Stress Relieving Diffuser Blend 4

Materials

- 4 drops grapefruit essential oil
- 2 drops jasmine essential oil
- 1 drop ylang ylang essential oil

Directions

Combine ingredients in your diffuser and use as instructed.

September 30

Stress Relieving Bath Oil

Materials
- ½ C rice bran oil
- 8 drops grapefruit essential oil
- 4 drops jasmine essential oil
- 3 drop ylang ylang essential oil

Directions

Combine all ingredients together in a glass bowl. Transfer mixture to a dark colored glass bottle. To use, add 1-2 tbsp to your bathwater.

What You need to Know about Using Essential Oils

When it comes to using essential oils, you really need to do your research to learn how to use them safely. There are many things you need to know about working with essential oils. So many, in fact, that it really requires full books on the subject. For the sake of space, we have listed the most important things that you need to know about working with essential oils for aromatherapy.

- Use Natural Products – If a product is labeled as "fragrance", "fragrance oil", or "perfume", it is not an essential oil. They are completely different things.
- Essential Oils are Natural – Because they are natural, they can't be patented, and therefore are never used in pharmaceutical drugs. They are mainly used by those who practice alternative forms of health care.
- Do Not Use Undiluted Oils on Skin – Most essential oils must be diluted before being applied to the skin. They must be used in combination with carrier oils, butters, waxes, etc. That being said, there are a few oils that can be used undiluted. These are lavender, German chamomile, sandalwood, and rose geranium.
- Do Not Use ANY Undiluted Oils on Children – It is extremely important that you never use any undiluted essential oils on preparations for babies and children. Do not even use the "safe" essential oils listed above. Children's skin is much more sensitive than adults' skin. Also, be sure to use half of the recommended amounts of essential oils when making recipes to use on children.
- Do Not Use these Essential Oils when Pregnant or Nursing – Aniseed, chamomile, cinnamon, clary sage, clove, ginger, cedarwood, lemon, jasmine, nutmeg, rosemary, and sage. Always speak with your physician before using essential oils during pregnancy or while nursing, and never use any essential oils during your first trimester.
- Be Careful of Food Allergies – Many essential oils are also used as flavors in foods. That being said, if you are allergic to certain foods, you will be allergic to the essential oils. For instance, if you can't eat turkey that has been cooked with thyme, avoid using thyme essential oil.
- Do a Skin Patch Test – Before using any essential oils in skin care products, it is a good idea to do a patch test to make sure that you aren't allergic to the oils. Mix a couple of drops of the essential oil with a tablespoon of carrier oil. Apply to the inside of your elbow, and wait 24 hours to see if there is a reaction. If there is no reaction, it is safe for you to use.
- Store Essential Oils in Dark Colored Glass Bottles – Essential oils lose their potency when exposed to light. Also make sure that they are stored in a dark cupboard.
- Essential Oils last for a Decade – As long as they are stored properly, essential oils can last for five to 10 years. Because you only use a few drops per recipe, a bottle will last for a very long time.

White Lemon

October

all is here, and it is time to start getting ready for the holiday season. This month, you will find loads of diffuser recipes that will make every room in your home smell amazing. There are also recipes for skin care products, body sprays, and much more. Be sure to check out the special apple/cinnamon Halloween recipes.

October 1

Aromatherapy Bath Salts

Materials

- 2 C Epsom salts
- 1 C coarse sea salt
- 15 drops rose essential oil
- 5 drops lavender essential oil
- 5 drops geranium essential oil

Directions

Combine all ingredients together in a glass bowl. Transfer mixture to an airtight container. To use, add ½ C of the mixture to your bathwater.

October 2

Aromatherapy Massage Oil

Materials

- 1 ounce rice bran oil
- 8 drops lemon essential oil
- 5 drops peppermint essential oil

Directions

Combine all ingredients together in a glass bowl. Transfer mixture to a dark colored glass bottle. To use, apply a few drops and massage gently.

October 3

Aromatherapy Soy Jar Candle

Materials

- 1 pound soy wax chips
- 20 drops green apple essential oil
- 10 drops apple essential oil
- Red candle dye
- Cotton wick
- Mason jars

Directions

Heat the jar in a pan of hot water. In a double boiler over medium heat, melt the soy wax chips and add candle dye. Remove from heat and let cool to 140 degrees F. Add essential oils and stir to blend. Pour mixture into Mason jars, slowly to keep mixture from splashing. Allow to completely harden before using.

October 4

Aromatherapy Hand Lotion

Materials

- 2 tbsp emulsifying wax
- ½ tsp stearic acid
- 1/3 C rice bran oil
- ½ C pure distilled water
- 1 tsp vitamin E oil
- 10 drops grapefruit seed extract
- 1 tbsp vegetable glycerin
- 15 drops lavender essential oil
- 5 drops rose essential oil

Directions

In a double boiler over medium heat, combine wax, rice bran oil, glycerin, and stearic acid. When ingredients have melted and blended together, remove from heat and add vitamin E oil. Slowly add the purified water, whisking until the mixture is an even color throughout. Add the essential oils and grapefruit seed extract. Transfer mixture to a clean plastic bottle. Shake well before each use.

October 5

Aromatherapy Facial Steam for Dry Skin

Materials

- 5 drops chamomile essential oil
- 5 drops rose essential oil
- 3 drops peppermint essential oil

Directions

Add essential oils to a bowl of boiling water. Lean over the bowl so your face is close, and cover your head and the bowl with a towel. Sit in this position for 5-10 minutes.

October 6

Aromatherapy Facial Steam for Normal Skin

Materials

- 5 drops geranium essential oil
- 5 drops jasmine essential oil
- 5 drops rose essential oil

Directions

Add essential oils to a bowl of boiling water. Lean over the bowl so your face is close, and cover your head and the bowl with a towel. Sit in this position for 5-10 minutes.

October 7

Aromatherapy Facial Steam for Oily Skin

Materials

- 5 drops jasmine essential oil
- 5 drops sandalwood essential oil
- 2 drops tea tree oil

Directions

Add essential oils to a bowl of boiling water. Lean over the bowl so your face is close, and cover your head and the bowl with a towel. Sit in this position for 5-10 minutes.

October 8

Aromatherapy Facial Steam for Sensitive Skin

Materials

- 5 drops chamomile essential oil
- 3 drops lavender essential oil
- 2 drops neroli essential oil

Directions

Add essential oils to a bowl of boiling water. Lean over the bowl so your face is close, and cover your head and the bowl with a towel. Sit in this position for 5-10 minutes.

October 9

Aromatherapy Facial Steam for Skin Conditions

Materials
- 6 drops lavender essential oil
- 4 drops chamomile essential oil
- 4 drops jasmine essential oil

Directions
Add essential oils to a bowl of boiling water. Lean over the bowl so your face is close, and cover your head and the bowl with a towel. Sit in this position for 5-10 minutes.

October 10

Aromatherapy Facial Scrub for Dry Skin

Materials
- 2 C rolled oats
- ½ C almonds
- ½ C powdered milk
- 4 drops frankincense essential oil
- 2 drops patchouli essential oil
- 2 drops sandalwood essential oil
- 2 drops chamomile essential oil
- 2 drops ylang ylang essential oil

Directions
Grind oats and almonds separately until they are both fine powders. Stir oat and almond powders together, and add the essential oils. Transfer mixture to an airtight container. To use, mix 1tbsp of the scrub mixture with enough lotion to make a sticky paste. Massage into skin and rinse with clear, warm water.

October 11

Aromatherapy Acne Face Scrub

Materials
- 2 C rolled oats
- ½ C corn meal
- ½ C kaolin clay
- 4 drops lemongrass essential oil

- 4 drops lavender essential oil
- 2 drops tea tree oil
- 2 drops rose geranium essential oil

Directions

Grind oats until they are a fine powder. Add the essential oils. Transfer mixture to an airtight container. To use, mix 1tbsp of the scrub mixture with enough lotion to make a sticky paste. Massage into skin and rinse with clear, warm water.

October 12

Aromatherapy Facial Mask for Dry Skin

Materials

- 2 tbsp kaolin clay
- 1 egg yolk
- ½ tsp raw honey
- ½ tsp apple cider vinegar
- 2 drops rose essential oil
- 1 drop neroli essential oil

Directions

In a small glass bowl, whisk together all ingredients except the kaolin clay. Add the clay, a little bit at a time, until you have created a smooth paste. To use, dampen skin and apply all over face, avoiding your eyes and mouth. Leave the mask on for 15-20 minutes. Rinse with clear, warm water.

October 13

Aromatherapy Facial Mask for Oily Skin

Materials

- 2 tbsp kaolin clay
- 2 tbsp low fat yogurt
- 2 drops lemongrass essential oil
- 1 drop tea tree oil

Directions

Combine all ingredients together in a glass bowl to create a paste. To use, dampen skin and apply all over face, avoiding your eyes and mouth. Leave the mask on for 15-20 minutes. Rinse with clear, warm water.

October 14

Aromatherapy Facial Mask for Normal Skin

Materials

- 1 tbsp kaolin clay
- 1 tsp low fat yogurt
- ½ tsp raw honey
- ¼ tsp jojoba oil
- 1 drop lavender essential oil
- 1 drop neroli essential oil

Directions

In a small glass bowl, whisk together all ingredients except the kaolin clay. Add the clay, a little bit at a time, until you have created a smooth paste. To use, dampen skin and apply all over face, avoiding your eyes and mouth. Leave the mask on for 15-20 minutes. Rinse with clear, warm water.

October 15

Aromatherapy Facial Mask for Sensitive Skin

Materials

- ½ tbsp. kaolin clay
- ½ tbsp. rolled oats
- ½ tsp avocado oil
- ½ tsp liquid aloe vera
- ½ tsp raw honey
- ½ tsp milk
- 1 drop chamomile essential oil
- 1 drop jasmine essential oil
- 1 drop lavender essential oil

Directions

Grind oats to a very fine powder. Whisk oil, honey, and aloe vera together. Slowly add the kaolin clay and oats, and mix until you have a smooth paste. To use, apply to damp skin on face, avoiding the eyes and mouth. Sit for 15-20 minutes. Rinse with clear, warm water.

October 16

Aromatherapy Cleanser for Normal Skin

Materials

- 1/3 C rose water
- 1/3 C rose geranium water
- 1 tbsp vegetable glycerin
- 1 drop rose geranium essential oil
- 1 drop ylang ylang essential oil

Directions

Combine all ingredients together in a glass bottle. Shake well before each use.

October 17

Aromatherapy Cleanser for Combination Skin

Materials

- ½ C lavender water
- 2 tbsp vegetable glycerin
- 2 tbsp aloe vera gel
- 4 drops lavender essential oil
- 4 drops petitgrain essential oil
- 2 drops rose geranium essential oil
- 1 drop ylang ylang essential oil

Directions

Combine all ingredients together in a glass bottle. Shake well before each use.

October 18

Aromatherapy Cleanser for Dry Skin

Materials

- ½ C lavender water
- 2 tbsp vegetable glycerin
- 2 tbsp aloe vera gel
- 4 drops palmarosa essential oil
- 4 drops frankincense essential oil
- 2 drops sandalwood essential oil
- 1 drop jasmine essential oil

Directions

Combine all ingredients together in a glass bottle. Shake well before each use.

October 19

Aromatherapy Cleanser for Oily Skin

Materials

- ½ C lavender water
- 2 tbsp vegetable glycerin
- 2 tbsp aloe vera gel
- 3 drops petitgrain essential oil
- 3 drops lemongrass essential oil
- 3 drops tea tree oil
- 1 drop chamomile essential oil

Directions

Combine all ingredients together in a glass bottle. Shake well before each use.

October 20

Olive Oil Facial Cleanser for Dry Skin

Materials

- ½ C extra virgin olive oil
- 5 drops sandalwood essential oil
- 5 drops patchouli essential oil
- 2 drops chamomile essential oil
- 2 drops geranium essential oil
- 1 drop jasmine essential oil

Directions

Combine all ingredients together in a dark colored glass bottle, let cure for 24 hours before using. To use, pour a small amount of cleanser into the palm of your hand and massage into skin. Soak a washcloth in hot water, and hold against your face until the cloth cools. Rinse with clear, cool water.

October 21

Olive Oil Facial Cleanser for Damaged Skin

Materials

- ½ C extra virgin olive oil
- 10 drops lavender essential oil
- 2 drops sandalwood essential oil
- 2 drops chamomile essential oil
- 1 drop rose essential oil

Directions

Combine all ingredients together in a dark colored glass bottle, let cure for 24 hours before using. To use, pour a small amount of cleanser into the palm of your hand and massage into skin. Soak a washcloth in hot water, and hold against your face until the cloth cools. Rinse with clear, cool water.

October 22

Olive Oil Facial Cleanser for Mature Skin

Materials

- ½ C extra virgin olive oil
- 4 drops sandalwood essential oil
- 4 drops frankincense essential oil
- 3 drops neroli essential oil
- 2 drops rose essential oil
- 2 drops palmarosa essential oil
- 1 drop helichrysum essential oil

Directions

Combine all ingredients together in a dark colored glass bottle, let cure for 24 hours before using. To use, pour a small amount of cleanser into the palm of your hand and massage into skin. Soak a washcloth in hot water, and hold against your face until the cloth cools. Rinse with clear, cool water.

October 23

Olive Oil Facial Cleanser for Sensitive Skin

Materials

- ½ C extra virgin olive oil
- 12 drops lavender essential oil

- 2 drops jasmine essential oil
- 1 drop vetiver essential oil

Directions

Combine all ingredients together in a dark colored glass bottle, let cure for 24 hours before using. To use, pour a small amount of cleanser into the palm of your hand and massage into skin. Soak a washcloth in hot water, and hold against your face until the cloth cools. Rinse with clear, cool water.

October 24

Olive Oil Facial Cleanser for Skin Conditions

Materials

- ½ C extra virgin olive oil
- 15 drops sandalwood essential oil
- 15 drops patchouli essential oil
- 2 drops palmarosa essential oil
- 2 drops helichrysum essential oil
- 1 drop chamomile essential oil

Directions

Combine all ingredients together in a dark colored glass bottle, let cure for 24 hours before using. To use, pour a small amount of cleanser into the palm of your hand and massage into skin. Soak a washcloth in hot water, and hold against your face until the cloth cools. Rinse with clear, cool water.

October 25

Olive Oil Facial Cleanser for Oily Skin

Materials

- ½ C extra virgin olive oil
- 5 drops tea tree oil
- 5 drops lemongrass essential oil
- 2 drops petitgrain essential oil
- 2 drops lemon essential oil
- 1 drop cedarwood essential oil
- 1 drop geranium essential oil

Directions

Combine all ingredients together in a dark colored glass bottle, let cure for 24 hours before using. To use, pour a small amount of cleanser into the palm of your hand and massage into skin. Soak a washcloth in hot water, and hold against your face until the cloth cools. Rinse with clear, cool water.

October 26

Olive Oil Facial Cleanser for Normal Skin

Materials

- ½ C extra virgin olive oil
- 5 drops lavender essential oil
- 5 drops orange essential oil
- 2 drops geranium essential oil
- 2 drops palmarosa essential oil
- 1 drop ylang ylang essential oil

Directions

Combine all ingredients together in a dark colored glass bottle, let cure for 24 hours before using. To use, pour a small amount of cleanser into the palm of your hand and massage into skin. Soak a washcloth in hot water, and hold against your face until the cloth cools. Rinse with clear, cool water.

October 27

Aromatherapy Halloween Body Spray

Materials

- 1 C pure distilled water
- 1/3 C witch hazel
- 10 drops apple essential oil
- 5 drops cinnamon essential oil

Directions

Combine all ingredients together in a spray bottle. Shake well before each use.

October 28

Halloween Diffuser Blend

Materials

- 3 drops apple essential oil
- 2 drops cinnamon essential oil
- 1 drop clove essential oil

Directions

Combine essential oils in your diffuser and use as instructed.

October 29

Candy Apple Diffuser Blend

Materials

- 3 drops apple essential oil
- 3 drops green apple essential oil

Directions

Combine essential oils in your diffuser and use as instructed.

October 30

Spicy Aromatherapy Body Spray

Materials

- ½ C pure distilled water
- ¼ C witch hazel
- 10 drops cinnamon essential oil
- 5 drops clove essential oil
- 3 drops cinnamon bark essential oil
- 2 drops nutmeg essential oil

Directions

Combine all ingredients together in a spray bottle. Shake well before each use.

October 31

Aromatherapy Facial Moisturizer

Materials

- 2 tbsp emulsifying wax
- 1/3 C rice bran oil
- 1 tbsp vegetable glycerin
- 1/3 C rose geranium water
- 1 tsp vitamin E oil
- 10 drops grapefruit seed extract
- 10 drops lavender essential oil
- 2 drops chamomile essential oil
- 1 drop palmarosa essential oil

Directions

In a double boiler over medium heat, combine the emulsifying wax, rice bran oil, and vegetable glycerin. When ingredients have melted and blended together, remove from heat and add vitamin E oil. In a separate double boiler, heat the rose geranium water to lukewarm. Pour water into the oil mixture, whisking until mixture becomes thick and creamy. Add the grapefruit seed extract and essential oils, and whisk to blend. Transfer mixture to a covered glass jar and store in a cool, dark place.

How to Use Aromatherapy in Your Bath

Aromatherapy has been used for hundreds of years to help people relax, revive themselves, have better concentration, and treat various health problems. One of the best ways to get the full effects of aromatherapy is to enjoy an aromatherapy bath. You get to enjoy a long, hot soak in the tub, while inhaling the healing vapors of the essential oils. But, there is a lot more to a true aromatherapy bath than just dumping some essential oils in the water. Read on to learn more.

Choosing the Right Essential Oils for Your Bath

The first step in the process of taking an aromatherapy bath is to choose the right essential oils. You can use single oils, or a combination of different oils for specific purposes. For instance, if you want softer skin, use a combination of lavender and rose essential oils. To treat congestion, use mint essential oils. It is a good idea to invest in a book about the uses for each type of essential oil so you can choose the best ones for aromatherapy baths.

Mix the Oils

Once you have chosen the essential oils for your aromatherapy bath, it is time to mix them. Make sure that they are mixed with a carrier oil, such as jojoba oil, sweet almond oil, or rice bran oil. A good ratio is to use one ounce of carrier oil with about 10 drops of essential oils (more if you prefer a stronger scent).

Draw Your Bath

Fill the tub with hot water, but not so hot that you won't be comfortable in the bath. If the aromatherapy bath is for a child, make sure that the water isn't too hot. Add some cold water if necessary. Add the essential oil mixture directly under the running water. This is going to help distribute it throughout the water better than just dumping the oils into the water after the bath has been drawn. Add a cup of whole milk to the water to help make your skin even softer.

Set the Mood

Before you get in the tub, it is time to set the mood for your relaxing aromatherapy bath. How you do this is completely up to you. Some suggestions include lighting a few candles (scented candles are best for even more aromatherapy), turning on your favorite music, and dimming the lights. If you are using a lot of candles, turn the lights off completely. Get the kids out of the house, and make sure you have at least 20 minutes to relax in the tub.

Prepare Your Skin

Before you get into the water, dry brush your skin to exfoliate it. This will help to increase your skin's circulation and remove dead skin cells. It will also make it easier for the essential oils to penetrate and moisturize the skin.

Take Your Aromatherapy Bath

Now it is time to step into the water and enjoy the luxury of an aromatherapy bath. Soak for 15-20 minutes to get the full effects of the essential oils. After getting out of the tub, wrap up in a big, warm towel for a few minutes, and then use your favorite moisturizer.

November

The holiday season is upon us, and that means that there is going to be loads of amazing smells in your home from the delicious foods you will be cooking. Why not add to those smells with some holiday scented aromatherapy room sprays? This month, you will find some terrific candle recipes with scents that will get you pumped for the holidays. Of course, there are also some great diffuser recipes, skin care recipes, and some household cleaners to help you get your home ready for holiday entertaining.

November 1

Thanksgiving Diffuser Blend 1

Materials

- 20 drops bergamot essential oil
- 10 drops grapefruit essential oil
- 10 drops cypress essential oil
- 10 drops frankincense essential oil
- 5 drops ylang ylang essential oil
- 2 drops ginger essential oil

Directions

Combine all ingredients together in a dark colored glass bottle. To use, add 5-6 drops to your diffuser and use as instructed.

November 2

Thanksgiving Diffuser Blend 2

Materials

- 4 drops cypress essential oil
- 3 drops pine essential oil
- 2 drops sandalwood essential oil

Directions

Combine essential oils in your diffuser and use as instructed.

November 3

Thanksgiving Diffuser Blend 3

Materials

- 2 drops cinnamon essential oil
- 2 drops clove essential oil
- 1 drop orange essential oil

Directions

Combine essential oils in your diffuser and use as instructed.

November 4

Thanksgiving Diffuser Blend 4

Materials

- 3 drops nutmeg essential oil
- 2 drops cinnamon essential oil
- 1 drop ginger essential oil

Directions

Combine essential oils in your diffuser and use as instructed.

November 5

Thanksgiving Diffuser Blend 5

Materials

- 3 drops pine essential oil
- 2 drops cedarwood essential oil
- 1 drop nutmeg essential oil

Directions

Combine essential oils in your diffuser and use as instructed.

November 6

Aromatherapy Holiday Air Spray 1

Materials

- 1 C pure distilled water
- 10 drops nutmeg essential oil
- 5 drops cinnamon essential oil

Directions

Combine ingredients together in a spray bottle. Shake well before each use.

November 7

Aromatherapy Holiday Air Spray 2

Materials

- 1 C pure distilled water
- 10 drops pumpkin essential oil
- 3 drops nutmeg essential oil
- 1 drop cinnamon essential oil

Directions

Combine ingredients together in a spray bottle. Shake well before each use.

November 8

Aromatherapy Holiday Air Spray 3

Materials

- 1 C pure distilled water
- 20 drops cinnamon essential oil

Directions

Combine ingredients together in a spray bottle. Shake well before each use.

November 9

Aromatic Napkins

Materials

- 5 drops pumpkin spice essential oil
- 3 drops nutmeg essential oil
- 2 drops ginger essential oil
- Cloth napkins

Directions

Combine essential oils together in a small glass bowl. Place a couple of drops of the essential oil mixture on each napkin. Place napkins in a plastic zip-lock bag, seal the bag, and allow to sit in a dark place for 24-48 hours.

November 10

Aromatic Tablecloth

Materials

- 10 drops pumpkin spice essential oil
- 6 drops nutmeg essential oil
- 4 drops ginger essential oil
- 2 drops clove essential oil
- Tablecloth
- 1 small square of cotton cloth

Directions

Wash tablecloth and place it in the dryer. Combine the essential oils in a small glass bowl, and soak the cotton cloth in the mixture. Place the cloth in the dryer with the tablecloth and dry as normal.

November 11

Holiday Bathroom Spray

Materials

- 1 ounce vodka
- 3-5 drops vegetable glycerin
- 15 drops sweet orange essential oil
- 10 drops clove bud essential oil
- ½ C pure distilled water

Directions

Combine all ingredients together in a spray bottle. Shake well before each use.

November 12

Cinnamon Toothpicks

Materials

- 1 box of 100 wooden toothpicks
- 30 drops cinnamon essential oil
- 1 tsp vodka
- 2 drops liquid Stevia

Directions

Combine ingredients together in a jar. Place toothpicks in the essential oil mixture, cover the jar, and let sit in a cool, dark place for at least two days. Shake the jar several times each day to make sure all of the toothpicks get fully saturated. Lay toothpicks out on a baking sheet for a couple of hours to dry.

November 13

Fresh Breath Spray

Materials

- ½ ounce vodka
- ½ ounce pure distilled water
- 1 tsp raw honey
- 2 drops liquid Stevia
- 15 drops cinnamon essential oil

Directions

Combine all ingredients together in a small spray bottle. Shake well before each use.

November 14

Holiday Dish Liquid

Materials

- 1 C liquid Castile soap
- 10 drops cinnamon essential oil
- 3 drops clove essential oil

Directions

Combine all ingredients together in a glass bowl. Transfer mixture to a clean dish liquid bottle.

November 15

Aromatherapy Gel Air Freshener

Materials

- 2 envelopes unflavored gelatin
- ½ C boiling water
- ½ C ice water

- 1 tbsp table salt
- 10 drops pumpkin essential oil
- 5 drops nutmeg essential oil
- 2 drops cinnamon essential oil
- Orange food grade colorant

Directions

Dissolve the gelatin in the boiling water. Add the ice water once all of the gelatin is completely dissolved. Add the essential oils, salt, and colorant. Pour mixture into prepared covered jars.

November 16

Aromatherapy Bath Melts

Materials

- ¼ C cocoa butter
- 2 tbsp sweet almond oil
- 20 drops lavender essential oil
- 5 drops lemon essential oil
- Food grade colorant (optional)

Directions

In a double boiler over medium heat, combine the cocoa butter and sweet almond oil. When ingredients have melted and blended together, remove from heat and add the essential oils. Pour mixture into prepared candy molds and allow to set.

November 17

Aromatherapy Sea Scent Bath Salts

Materials

- ½ C Epsom salts
- ½ C coarse sea salt
- 5 drops lavender essential oil
- 5 drops rose essential oil
- 2 drops chamomile essential oil
- Food grade colorant (optional)

Directions

Combine all ingredients together in a glass bowl. Transfer mixture to an airtight container. To use, add ½ C of the mixture to your bathwater.

November 18

Aromatherapy Solid Perfume

Materials

- 1 heaping tbsp grated beeswax
- 3 tbsp jojoba oil
- Liquid from 1 vitamin E capsule
- 40 drops lavender essential oil
- 40 drops rose essential oil
- 20 drops geranium essential oil

Directions

In a double boiler over medium heat, combine the beeswax and jojoba oil. When ingredients have melted and blended together, remove from heat. Allow mixture to cool for a few minutes, and add the vitamin E oil and essential oils. Pour mixture into prepared lip balm tubs or jars.

November 19

Aromatherapy Fizzy Bath Salts

Materials

- ¼ C baking soda
- 2 tbsp citric acid
- ¾ C sea salt
- 20 drops lemon essential oil
- 5 drops peppermint essential oil

Directions

Combine all ingredients together in a glass bowl. Transfer mixture to an airtight container. To use, add ½ C of the mixture to your bathwater.

November 20

Aromatherapy Linen Spritzer

Materials

- 2 C pure distilled water
- 2 tbsp rubbing alcohol
- 15 drops lavender essential oil

Directions

Combine all ingredients together in a spray bottle. Shake well before each use.

November 21

Aromatherapy Hot and Cold Pack

Materials

- Cotton fabric
- Whole flax seeds
- ½ C dried peppermint leaves
- 3-4 drops peppermint essential oil

Directions

Cut two 8" X 18" rectangles out of the cloth, and stitch three sides together. Fill the bag with flax seeds and dried herbs. Soak a cotton ball with peppermint essential oils, and place in the middle of the seeds and herbs. Stitch the top seam shut.

November 22

Aromatherapy Bubble Bath 1

Materials

- 1 ½ C liquid Castile soap
- 2 tbsp vegetable glycerin
- 1 tsp white sugar
- 5 drops lavender essential oil
- 4 drops lemon essential oil
- 1 drop chamomile essential oil

Directions

Combine all ingredients together in a glass bowl, stirring gently to blend without creating bubbles. Transfer mixture to a pump bottle.

November 23

Aromatherapy Bubble Bath 2

Materials

- 1 ½ C liquid Castile soap
- 2 tbsp vegetable glycerin
- 1 tsp white sugar
- 5 drops bergamot essential oil
- 4 drops orange essential oil
- 1 drop jasmine essential oil

Directions

Combine all ingredients together in a glass bowl, stirring gently to blend without creating bubbles. Transfer mixture to a pump bottle.

November 24

Aromatherapy Bubble Bath 3

Materials

- 1 ½ C liquid castile soap
- 2 tbsp vegetable glycerin
- 1 tsp white sugar
- 5 drops lavender essential oil
- 4 drops sandalwood essential oil
- 1 drop clove essential oil

Directions

Combine all ingredients together in a glass bowl, stirring gently to blend without creating bubbles. Transfer mixture to a pump bottle.

November 25

Aromatherapy Bubble Bath 4

Materials

- 1 ½ C liquid castile soap
- 2 tbsp vegetable glycerin
- 1 tsp white sugar
- 10 drops vanilla essential oil

Directions

Combine all ingredients together in a glass bowl, stirring gently to blend without creating bubbles. Transfer mixture to a pump bottle.

November 26

Aromatherapy Bubble Bath 5

Materials

- 1 ½ C liquid Castile soap
- 2 tbsp vegetable glycerin
- 1 tsp white sugar
- 3 drops rose absolute essential oil
- 2 drops palmarosa essential oil
- 1 drop rose geranium essential oil

Directions

Combine all ingredients together in a glass bowl, stirring gently to blend without creating bubbles. Transfer mixture to a pump bottle.

November 27

Aromatherapy Citrus Body Butter

Materials

- 2/3 C shea butter
- 1/3 C mango butter
- 1 tsp jojoba oil
- 3 tsp grapeseed oil
- 8 drops bergamot essential oil
- 8 drops lemongrass essential oil
- 6 drops palmarosa essential oil
- 2 drops cypress essential oil
- 1 drop rose geranium essential oil
- 1 tsp corn starch
- 1 tsp cosmetic mica to make the mixture shimmer

Directions

In a double boiler over medium heat, combine the shea butter, mango butter, jojoba oil, and grapeseed oil. When ingredients have melted and blended together, remove from heat and add the corn starch, mica, and essential oils. Transfer mixture to prepared jars with covers.

November 28

Aromatherapy Acne Cream

Materials

- 1 tbsp emulsifying wax
- 1 tbsp aloe vera gel
- 1/3 C witch hazel
- 4 tsp grapeseed oil
- ½ tsp stearic acid
- ½ tsp vitamin E oil
- 5 drops grapefruit seed extract
- 5 drops lavender essential oil
- 3 drops lemon essential oil
- 1 drop rose essential oil

Directions

In a double boiler over medium heat, combine oil, emulsifying wax, and stearic acid. Heat the witch hazel to lukewarm in a separate double boiler. Slowly add the warmed witch hazel to the wax mixture, whisking constantly. Add the grapefruit seed extract and essential oils, and continue whisking until mixture is thick and creamy. Transfer mixture to covered jars.

November 29

Aromatherapy Mirror Cleaner

Materials

- 1 ½ C white vinegar
- ½ C pure distilled water
- 10 drops lemon essential oil

Directions

Combine all ingredients together in a spray bottle. Shake well before each use.

November 30

Aromatherapy Face Brightening Toner

Materials

- ½ C lemon juice
- 2/3 C witch hazel

White Lemon

- 1 C pure distilled water
- 2 drops tea tree oil

Directions

Combine all ingredients together in a glass bowl. Transfer mixture to a dark colored glass bottle. Use as you would your regular skin toner.

Aromatherapy around Your Home

There are all kinds of ways that you can get the benefits of aromatherapy. One is to make special cleaning products to use in your home. Not only will your home smell wonderful, the aromas will also offer added health benefits. Let's take a look at the many ways you can use aromatherapy around your home.

- Underwear Drawers – You can freshen your underwear by putting a few drops of essential oils on a couple of cotton balls, and placing the cotton balls in the drawers. Recommended scents include rose, jasmine, ylang ylang, lavender, and geranium. Choose your favorite scents, because your clothes are going to absorb them.
- No More Air Fresheners – Instead of using commercially-prepared air fresheners that are loaded with chemicals and artificial scents, place a few drops of essential oils on cotton balls and place them around your home. Use different scents in each room.
- Simmer Some Spices – While you are cooking, you can neutralize the strong odors simply by simmering water and adding a few drops of essential oils to the water. Recommended oils for odor neutralization include cinnamon, clove, and cardamom.
- Vacuum Fresh Scents – Before you vacuum the carpets, spray a piece of tissue paper with 2 drops of mandarin essential oil and 2 drops of lemon essential oil. Let the vacuum cleaner suck up the tissue, and as you vacuum the carpets, the scent will be released.
- Give it a Mist – Fill a spray bottle with a cup of pure distilled water and 15-20 drops of your favorite essential oils. Spray a mist around the room whenever you want a nice, fresh scent. Recommended essential oils include pine, lemon, and eucalyptus.
- Freshen Your Cupboards – Add a few drops of essential oils to cotton balls and place them inside your kitchen cupboards to keep them smelling nice and fresh. Recommended essential oils for this include bergamot, lavender, cedarwood, and lime.
- Get Rid of Pet Odors – Add 10-15 drops of essential oil to a half a bucket of hot water and the cleanser you normally use. Use this solution to mop the areas where the pet odors are the worst. For carpeting, mix the essential oils in a spray bottle and spritz the carpets. Recommended essential oils include lemon, eucalyptus, geranium, and lemongrass.
- Refresh Your Carpets – Combine ¾ C baking soda with 10 drops of lemon essential oil. Store in an airtight container for 2 days, and then sprinkle onto carpets. Leave mixture on the carpets for 3-4 hours, and then vacuum.
- Freshen Up Your Laundry – Cut a square of cotton fabric and add a few drops of your favorite essential oils. Place the cloth in the dryer with your laundry for a clean, fresh scent. Citrus and floral essential oils are ideal for this purpose.
- Make Closets and Wardrobes Smell Great – Mix 2 drops of lavender essential oil, geranium essential oil, and basil essential oil in a small glass bowl. Place this mixture on a cotton ball and place it in a closet or wardrobe.

December

It is holiday time, and it's the season for giving gifts that come from the heart. What could be more heartfelt than a gift you make yourself? Your friends and family members will love aromatherapy gifts that have been made specifically with them in mind. So, we are devoting this month to awesome aromatherapy recipes for gifts you can give to everyone on your gift list.

December 1

Holiday Scented Coasters

Materials

- Pre-cut, coaster-sized wood shapes
- Red and green felt
- Battery-operated diffuser pads
- 10 drops peppermint essential oil
- Glue gun and glue

Directions

Cut two pieces of felt to fit over pre-cut wood shapes and diffuser pads. You can cut extra felt in the shape of trees and other holiday decorations to glue on the top. Glue one piece of felt to a piece of wood, and glue a diffuser pad on top of the felt. On the second piece of felt, cut a hole in the center. Glue it on top of the diffuser pad. Place the decorations on this piece of felt, being careful not to cover the hole. Add the essential oils to the hole.

December 2

Aromatherapy Holiday Air Fresheners

Materials

- 1 ounce pure distilled water
- 30 drops pine essential oil
- Small, dark colored, decorative bottle with a cover
- Ribbon and gift tag

Directions

Combine ingredients in the bottle. Attach gift tag with ribbon.

December 3

Aromatherapy Bath Salts Gift Boxes

Materials

- 1 C Epsom Salts
- 1 C coarse sea salt
- 10 drops peppermint essential oil
- 5 drops pine essential oil
- Green food grade colorant

- Small gift boxes

Directions

Combine salts, essential oils, and colorant in a glass bowl. Transfer contents to gift boxes.

December 4

Aromatherapy Tea Candles

Materials

- 6 tbsp grated beeswax
- 2 candle wicks
- 2 small glass candle holders
- 35 drops peppermint essential oil
- Red candle dye
- Ribbons

Directions

In a double boiler over medium heat, melt the beeswax. Remove from heat and add the peppermint essential oil and candle dye. Fill candle holders half way, and let mixture begin to solidify. Add the wicks and fill the candle holders the rest of the way. Decorate with pretty ribbons.

December 5

Aromatherapy Ornaments

Materials

- 2 glass ball ornaments
- 2 flat, checker-sized pieces of wood, painted to match glass ball ornaments
- Aroma testing strips
- 10 drops pine essential oil
- 10 drops peppermint essential oil

Directions

Remove top pieces from glass ball ornaments. Glue the flat pieces of wood to the bottom of both ornaments. Now they have a base so they will sit upright. Add pine essential oil to one ornament, and peppermint essential oil to the other. Create a small stack of aroma test strips, one on top of the other. Slide this stack inside the ornament far enough so they touch the essential oils. Spread the tops of the strips outwards to resemble a fan.

December 6

Holiday Spritzer

Materials

- ½ tsp pure distilled water
- 5 drops peppermint essential oil
- 1 pinch Epsom salts
- 3ml spray bottle

Directions

Combine all ingredients together in the spray bottle. Add a ribbon and a gift tag.

December 7

Aromatherapy Stationery Paper

Materials

- 5-10 sheets of paper
- 10 drops cinnamon essential oil
- 3 drops frankincense essential oil
- 2 drops myrhh essential oil
- Facial tissue
- Zip-lock baggie

Directions

Fold the piece of facial tissue into eighths. Blend the essential oils, and sprinkle the blend onto the tissue. Place the tissue between the sheets of paper. Place the entire bundle inside the baggie, seal, and let sit for a couple of days in a cool, dark place. Package the paper in a nice gift box.

December 8

Aromatherapy Stationery Envelopes

Materials

- 5-10 sheets of paper
- 5 drops cinnamon essential oil
- 1 drop frankincense essential oil
- 1 drop myrhh essential oil
- Facial tissue
- Zip-lock baggie

Directions

Fold the piece of facial tissue into eights. Blend the essential oils, and sprinkle the blend onto the tissue. Place the tissue between the envelopes. Place the entire bundle inside the baggie, seal, and let sit for a couple of days in a cool, dark place. Package the envelopes with the paper in a nice gift box.

December 9

Aromatherapy Soap for Kids

Materials

- 1 pound clear glycerin melt and pour soap base
- 1 tbsp liquid aloe vera
- 5-6 drops cinnamon essential oil
- Red food grade colorant
- Silver food grade glitter
- Kids' soap molds

Directions

In a double boiler over medium heat, combine the glycerin soap base and aloe vera. When soap base has melted, remove from heat and add the cinnamon essential oil, colorant, and glitter. Pour into prepared soap molds and allow to sit for a couple of hours to harden (or place in the freezer for ½ hour).

December 10

Kids' Bath Fizzies

Materials

- 10 tbsp baking soda
- 10 tsp citric acid
- 50 drops grapefruit essential oil
- 50 drops sweet orange essential oil
- Food grade colorant (optional)
- Spray bottle with water

Directions

Mix baking soda and citric acid in a glass bowl. Add the essential oils and colorant. If the mixture is too dry, spritz with a bit of water. Pack mixture tightly into prepared molds. Allow to dry for 24-48 hours.

December 11

Aromatherapy Finger Paints

Materials

- ¼ C liquid laundry starch
- 5 drops food coloring
- Essential oil to match color of food coloring (eg. Lemon = yellow, cherry = red, etc.)
- 2 ounce paint bottle

Directions

Combine all ingredients together in a small glass bowl. Transfer mixture to paint bottle. Repeat process for different colors and scents.

December 12

Lavender-Scented Pillow

Materials

- Small, decorative pillow
- Essential oils aroma pad
- 20 drops lavender essential oil
- Needle and thread

Directions

Stitch the aroma pad to the front of the pillow. Add the essential oils to the aroma pad. Include a small vial of essential oils with this gift so the recipient can replenish the aroma.

December 13

Aromatherapy Lip Balm for Kids

Materials

- 2 tbsp grated beeswax
- 1 tbsp cocoa butter
- 3 tbsp jojoba oil
- 10 drops peppermint essential oil

Directions

In a double boiler over medium heat, combine the beeswax, cocoa butter, and jojoba oil. When ingredients have melted and blended together, remove from heat and add the peppermint essential oil. Pour into prepared lip balm tubes or tubs.

December 14

Aromatherapy Pomander

Materials

- 1 large orange
- Whole cloves
- 3-4 drops clove essential oil
- ¼" ribbon
- Straight pins with decorative ball heads

Directions

Soak ribbon in peppermint essential oil and allow to dry. Place ribbon around orange in a criss-cross pattern, holding in place with the straight pins (leave ends long enough to tie a bow for hanging). Poke whole cloves into the open spaces between the ribbons on the orange.

December 15

Holiday Pillar Candle

Materials

- 1 pound grated beeswax
- 20 drops sweet orange essential oil
- 10 drops clove essential oil
- 5 drops cinnamon essential oil
- Red and green candle dye
- Long candle wick
- Empty cardboard milk carton
- Skewer

Directions

In a double boiler over medium heat, melt half of the beeswax. Do the same with the rest of the beeswax in a second double boiler. When wax has melted, remove from heat and add red colorant to one, green to the other. Blend the essential oils and add half to each mixture. Tie the end of the wick around the skewer. Cut the top off the milk carton, and place the skewer on top so the wick hangs down in the center. Begin pouring wax mixtures, allowing each layer to harden a bit before adding the next so you have red and green stripes. Allow to harden overnight, and peel away milk carton.

December 16

Scented Bubble Lotion

Materials

- ¾ C pure distilled water
- ¼ C liquid Castile soap or unscented dish liquid
- 1 tbsp vegetable glycerin
- 20 drops raspberry essential oil
- Empty bubble bottle and wand

Directions

Mix all ingredients together in the empty bubble bottle. To use, dip wand into mixture and blow big bubbles.

December 17

Shiny Lip Gloss

Materials

- 3 grams grated beeswax
- 5 grams cocoa butter
- 5 tsp jojoba oil
- Liquid from 1 vitamin E capsule
- 8 drops lavender essential oil
- 2 drops lemon essential oil

Directions

In a glass bowl, combine beeswax, cocoa butter, and jojoba oil. Heat in the microwave in 30-second increments. When ingredients have melted and blended together, add the vitamin E and essential oils. Pour mixture into prepared lip balm tubs or tubes.

December 18

Children's Monster Remover Spray

Materials

- ½ C pure distilled water

- 10 drops peppermint essential oil
- 5 drops spearmint essential oil
- 5 drops lemon essential oil

Directions

Combine all ingredients together in a spray bottle. Use at bedtime to ward off monsters in the closet and under the bed.

December 19

Candle Wick Diffusers

Materials

- 40 drops sweet orange essential oil
- 15 drops clove essential oil
- 2 small, dark colored glass bottles (dropper bottles are perfect for this project)
- 2 oil lamp wicks

Directions

Remove the droppers from the bottles, leaving the rubber nubs in place. Cut half of the rubber nubs off. Push wicks through the rubber nubs, and fray the top ends. Combine the essential oils, and put half of the mixture in each bottle. Replace the caps with the frayed wicks sticking out.

December 20

Holiday Body Spray

Materials

- 1 C pure distilled water
- ½ C witch hazel
- 25 drops sweet orange essential oil
- 10 drops clove essential oil
- 5 drops cinnamon essential oil
- 3 drops ginger essential oil

Directions

Combine all ingredients together in a spray bottle. Shake well before each use.

December 21

Spicy Diffuser Blend

Materials

- 3 drops clove essential oil
- 2 drops cinnamon essential oil
- 2 drops nutmeg essential oil
- 1 drop ginger essential oil

Directions

Combine essential oils in your diffuser and use as instructed.

December 22

Candy Cane Diffuser Blend

Materials

- 5 drops peppermint essential oil
- 3 drops spearmint essential oil

Directions

Combine essential oils in your diffuser and use as instructed.

December 23

Crystal Air Freshener

Materials

- 2 C coarse rock salt
- 40 drops frankincense essential oil
- 10 drops rose essential oil
- 10 drops ylang ylang essential oil
- 10 drops vanilla essential oil
- 1 tsp grain alcohol
- Food grade colorant (optional)
- Decorative glass containers

Directions

Blend the essential oils with the grain alcohol in a small glass bowl. Set aside. In a larger bowl, combine the coarse rock salt with essential oil blend and colorant. Fill glass containers with the mixture.

December 24

Essential Oils Sampler Pack

Materials

- 5-10 small bottles of essential oils
- Make-up bag with elastics to hold bottles in place
- Description cards

Directions

Print up description cards with information about each essential oil, and a recipe to use with each oil. Place bottles in the bag, and add the description cards.

December 25

Aromatherapy Exfoliating Foot Scrub

Materials

- ¼ C coarse sea salt
- ¼ C sweet almond oil
- 20 drops lemon essential oil

Directions

Combine all ingredients together in a glass bowl. Transfer mixture to an airtight container, and label as a gift.

December 26

Holiday Diffuser Blend 1

Materials

- 30 drops Douglas fir essential oil
- 15 drops cypress essential oil
- 20 drops orange essential oil
- 10 drops nutmeg essential oil

Directions

Combine all ingredients together in a dark colored glass bottle. To use, add 5-6 drops to your diffuser and use as instructed.

December 27

Holiday Diffuser Blend 2

Materials

- 40 drops cinnamon essential oil
- 40 drops orange essential oil
- 20 drops vanilla essential oil
- 15 drops nutmeg essential oil

Directions

Combine all ingredients together in a dark colored glass bottle. To use, add 5-6 drops to your diffuser and use as instructed.

December 28

Holiday Diffuser Blend 3

Materials

- 20 drops fir needle essential oil
- 20 drops tangerine essential oil
- 5 drops pine essential oil
- 5 drops star anise essential oil

Directions

Combine all ingredients together in a dark colored glass bottle. To use, add 5-6 drops to your diffuser and use as instructed.

December 29

Holiday Diffuser Blend 4

Materials

- 15 drops ginger essential oil
- 12 drops basil essential oil
- 20 drops lime essential oil
- 2 drops may chang essential oil

Directions

Combine all ingredients together in a dark colored glass bottle. To use, add 5-6 drops to your diffuser and use as instructed.

December 30

Holiday Diffuser Blend 5

Materials

- 15 drops mandarin essential oil
- 12 drops bay leaf essential oil
- 5 drops cinnamon essential oil
- 5 drops ginger essential oil

Directions

Combine all ingredients together in a dark colored glass bottle. To use, add 5-6 drops to your diffuser and use as instructed.

December 31

Holiday Diffuser Blend 6

Materials

- 15 drops myrrh essential oil
- 15 drops frankincense essential oil
- 30 drops sweet orange essential oil

Directions

Combine all ingredients together in a dark colored glass bottle. To use, add 5-6 drops to your diffuser and use as instructed.

White Lemon

Conclusion

We hope you have enjoyed trying out the 365 Aromatherapy Recipes for 365 Days. Now that you have the hang of working with essential oils, you can start creating your own recipes for diffuser blends, skin care products, novelty items, and so much more. Make sure that you keep all of the most-used essential oils on hand, so you can create any time the mood hits, or if you need to use aromatherapy for a quick pick-me-up. There is so much you can do with aromatherapy, and hopefully, we have put the bee in your bonnet to keep working on new projects.

Made in the USA
Lexington, KY
14 August 2017